IRB: Transforming Fear Into Love

For gifts and IRB Transforming Fear Into Love Experiences, go to bit.ly/XimenaDuqueValencia_IRB

I would like to subscribe and receive my free gift: bit.ly/IRB_PeaceMeditation

® IRB: Transforming Fear Into Love
Indigo Ray Balancing®
Ximena Duque Valencia
(All Rights Reserved)

ISBN-13: 978-1537678351
ISBN-10: 1537678353

Edit: Koradi S.A.S.
Calle 106B # 23-17 Int. 203
Bogotá – Colombia
Tel. (571) 2130845 - (57) 320 2056007 - (57) 320 2819419
E-mail: info@koradi.co, ximena@koradi.co

Translation to English by: Maëlle Jayet, www.mincor.net
Cover design and illustrations: Astrid Murillo Aristizábal
Design and layout: Janeth Albarracín G.

If this book has piqued your interest and you wish to be informed of all our activities, contact us through:
Facebook: bit.ly/XimenaDuqueValencia_IRB
YouTube: bit.ly/XimenaDuqueValenciaYouTube

All rights reserved. No part of this publication, including the cover design, may be reproduced, stored, transmitted or used in any way by any means, electronic, mechanical, optical, recording or electrographic, without the prior written consent of the publisher or the author. Go to bit.ly/XimenaDuqueValencia_IRB
if you wish to copy or scan any part of this book.

Contents

Acknowledgments VI

Introduction IX

My Beginning 11

Part One: The End of the Old

Chapter I. 25
2012: The Transition to the New Galactic Dawn

Chapter II. 29
The Key is Light

Chapter III. 31
Awakening

Chapter IV. 35
The Master Key

Chapter V. 45
Evolution

Chapter VI. 51
Inter-dimensionality

Chapter VII. 61
Critical Mass

Chapter VIII..69
Teachers or Gods?

Chapter IX...79
Where Are We Going?

Chapter X.°..83
The Original Pattern

Chapter XI...93
We Are One — Namaste —

Chapter XII...103
IRB, a Quantum Leap, an Existential Leap

Chapter XIII..113
Your Selection

PART TWO: THE CONVENTIONAL

Chapter XIV...119
Everything is Energy

Chapter XV...129
Cellular Memory

Chapter XVI...141
The Power of Belief

Chapter XVII..147
The Importance of the Heart

Part Three: IRB and DNA

Chapter XVII.. 155
The Alchemical Transmutation of Consciousness to Real Life and Purpose

Chapter XIX. 185
The Zero Point Field

Chapter XX 189
The Vehicles of Transformation

Chapter XXI. 233
The Concepts

Chapter XXII....255
The Four Pillars of Activation

Chapter XXIII...265
Transcending Paradigms

Epilogue..281

Appendix 282

Glossary..287

References 301

Acknowledgments

There have been so many wonderful people who have crossed my path and contributed to who I am, that naming them would take far too long. It is with thanks to all of them that I have written this book with the aim of contributing another spark of consciousness to the human race, to which I have decided to dedicate my time and energy. I thank you all, for within each of you exists a teacher who reflects my growth, my changes, my understanding of All that is, and my Love as the fundamental force of being One.

I give endless thanks to my patients for trusting me and placing their lives, healing, and joy in my hands; for allowing me to be their instrument of self-healing; and for growing through them a little more each day.

Thanks to Koradi for being the vessel through which I have been able to be known to the world and so reach so many wonderful people who have trusted in us; for making room for the new race that now populates the planet; and for helping us connect with undecipherable transparency.

To all those who trust that this is more than a book; it is a life project.

To Astrid, for saying, "Yes, one day…" for printing the beautiful art and for putting my thoughts on paper so that the world may enjoy it through the color and magic that we still have a hard time believing we possess; for making everything she touches beautiful, including the cover of the current edition; and for illustrating the channeling of Layer Thirteen and the logo of this splendid philosophy.

To Sergio Mejía and Santiago Mejía, wizards of music, for carrying the tune in perfect metric measure to the melody that makes it possible for the sixty-four codes of our DNA to activate Layer Thirteen. The thirteenth layer of our DNA plays the role of fundamental director in this orchestra that is capable of anything. And for providing, without limit, their rhythm and knowledge so that the music and mantras of IRB may always come with that harmonious touch that brings out the magic and meditative aspect.

To my daughter Kmi (Camila), for being the most important teacher in my life, for having taught me to let go and to uproot the unchanging, and the understanding of how To Be versus being somewhere, that love manifests in infinite ways, and that, in Love, anything is possible.

To Daniel, my "Viejo," who taught me humility, patience, art and Love in its purest form; to Ines, my mother, for teaching me that without discipline we cannot achieve our goals, and for allowing me to observe in her life the greatest example so that I could make another path for myself; without them and their teachings, their genes would not be in my DNA and my readers would not be reading any of this.

To my sisters, Patricia, María del Pilar, and Adriana, who complete the patchwork; each one, with their great differences, teaches me the powerful message that in respecting diversity we find Truth.

To Roger, my companion on this path, my soulmate, my light, my incentive to share the air, my everything: thank you for being the tireless accomplice who gives life to each of my crazy ideas, wishes, and projects; for being a most powerful wizard, a leader who touches all those that come into his life, and for being such a fundamental part of IRB and the universe's DNA!

To Janeth Albarracín García, for her easy-going personality, professionalism and exquisite mastery of the art of layout and design.

To Julio Mateus, whose proofreading and care will allow for an easier understanding of the following pages, as well as the reach of these words into the DNA, the genetic code, of each reader.

To Consuelo Acosta for believing in this project from the beginning, for her dedication and energy and infinite Love for each detail, and for effectively coordinating this project so that it could be brought to light impeccably.

I give thanks to Erica Vanina Cavallini, businesswoman and editor of topics relating to the transcendence of independence and the abundance of woman and family, and owner of Mujer Íntegra - www.mujerintegra.com

And finally, though I know there is an endless list of names not written here, to you, dear reader, for being interested in growing and, by reading this, assuming your responsibility as a vital part of All, to be a part of Love, wherever you may be in this limitless universe where anything is possible.

Introduction

This book is dedicated to humanity. It is meant for everyone who is looking for a change in their perspective toward life, to move forward in Love and Unity, and to free themselves of old paradigms that have kept them in a prison that cannot be seen, for its bars are made of fear and lack.

In the following pages, you will find a summary of numerous professional investigations, not only of a historical nature but also scientific and spiritual, that allow us to access a powerful tool for life, to support any purpose that is inherent to our existence from a point of Love and complete Consciousness, and to obtain the results that we have always wished for and many times have labeled as impossible.

This is not about some healing technique or a new dogma, nor is it more information to add to the mind's hard-drive. It is a project that may offer us immense transcendence, from a new concept of education, to flow with the purest of essences into all lifeforms.

My Beginning

*It is the same God, though there are many names;
you must choose one to call Him.*
Paulo Coelho

A few years ago, I learned that it is important to not speak in the first person, which empowers the ego. Even though it was quite difficult for me not to, as I was born in the same type of environment as was a great percentage of the human race, which is to say one of competition, individualism and self-importance. Though I tried hard to avoid first person, it rarely came out naturally. Now I understand that, aside from giving power to the ego, when we speak in first person it separates us from Source and the rest of those divine sparks that make up the universal reality that We Are One.

Furthermore, I have been speaking with a series of words and arguments that, surely, I would not have consciously used when speaking of my knowledge of the Third Density (or Third Dimension), which we will now refer to as 3D. I understand now that I am not speaking for myself but that it speaks through me. That is not to say that I am channeling some supernatural being, nor that I am the bringer of some message from some angel; it just means that Source consciousness is manifested through my meditations. But it may also manifest through you, who reads this book, as I am sure that it will divide your earthly existence into two: each written word helps you take a quantum leap into the evolution of consciousness for which you have been waiting for years, to remember who you truly are.

If I talk about "me" or "us," it comes back to the same idea, that we are all connected through an electromagnetic net that allows us to be part of a fundamental system that maintains the Earth's balance which itself is part of a perfect system that balances the millions of universes that exist in the All. This is why sometimes you will hear me say "I" and at other times "we;" it is all the same.

After many years of having wanted to do it, in 2012 I began to write this book. I am known for quickly achieving things once I've made up my mind to do them, so I always wondered why, if I longed to divulge that which I knew and considered important, my "saboteur" would appear each time I sat down to write even the first chapter. Well, today I can say with confidence that everything happens with perfect timing, one that deviates from the linearity with which the "elite" have wished to manipulate us through their established institutions all over this marvelous planet, the university of the human race, with the intention of separating us.

That is why I now understand that time is not a lineal manipulation. Everything converges simultaneously in a marvelous quantum ocean where anything is possible, and 2012 was the perfect year to shape a ripe new concept, decanted through in-depth research and experiments among my most loved ones; in other words, that which is captured in this book is verifiable, is true, and is as simple as Love, Living Light and Truth, which allow us all to be the architects and designers of our existence starting from the great teacher that is Our Consciousness, which can be updated every year, depending on our level of consciousness; that is, inevitably and always in the process of evolution.

My Beginning

The design of the human being has been greatly talked about, and there have been a great many discussions throughout the history of our civilizations about the existence of a grand creator of all that is, or perhaps a joint effort of many creators and gods. Either way, the point is not to get into the politics of religions or governments, though it will be necessary to touch lightly upon these topics. The primary and ultimate aim of this book is to help us understand truly that, whoever the Great Creator is, He did everything perfectly; which means without limits or illness or lack or resentment. There need be no negative feelings, poverty, nor a plethora of "teachers" pressuring us century after century, forcing us into debates that bring us to the same conclusions that prohibit permanent solutions to urgent questions about the supreme and divine energy that is ourselves, without exception.

In trying to remember when my obsession with these mysteries began, I have been brought to memories of my childhood, when instead of reading *Little Red Riding Hood,* I found *The Book of the Dead*, an Egyptian text that talks about the soul's rebirth and that death is not the end of who we are but simply the release of our physical body to give room to rebirth. That is why many have called it "crossing to the other side," a metaphor that brings us to the understanding that death is nothing more than a rebirth, starting again once we cross over. To give you an idea, this book has approximately two hundred chapters; such was the size of the book that obsessed me at nine years of age.

I later became immersed in the magic and poetry of Kahlil Gibran, a Lebanese artist and the author of *The Prophet*. I was equally passionate about texts written by Lobsang Rampa, such as: *Tibetan Sage, The Third Eye, Doctor from Lhasa, The Rampa Story, The Silver Cord, Living with the Lama, You Forever, The Saffron Robe*, and many other titles that carpeted the world of spirituality, the unknown, eternity, and the beyond. At that young age, I was already questioning an existence without any objective besides being born, reproducing, growing old and then dying. I did not dream of being married and having children, but of being able to contact a UFO and ask many things that perhaps beings in that strange vessel knew and I did not.

Among my favorite toys, besides Barbie dolls, were beautiful stones and crystals of different colors that I felt spoke to me. I felt them vibrate; they became dull when I was sad; they would appear in odd places; they would be lost then found again, as if trying to get my attention. Not wanting to be classified as crazy by adults, I tried to pretend that these voices were imaginary friends, and I became an expert at scripting childhood games that combined all sorts of unusual stories that I now understand were just sparks of memories of who I truly am.

To shorten an otherwise long life story and go directly into the new information about perfect co-creating from consciousness, I must skip various years, as does the Bible with Jesus, but without omitting the most important facts, as does the sacred book in skipping over aspects of Jesus's deep encounter with himself, his self-mastery, and his Divinity.

I got lost in the noise of the 3D world and was distracted from my mission, perhaps not unlike you or many others reading this book, who too have been afraid of this sacred encounter. Perhaps I should have prepared myself by having many points of view to understand the completeness that envelops the complexity yet simplicity of our bodies, minds, emotions, and the Universal Spirit that moves it all.

While lost, I met many wonderful people who instilled in me the curiosity to always go farther, and as I did not define myself by the path I had chosen from the *bardo* of my Atma transition, there was a climactic moment when the universe spoke to me and said, "If you have not heard me whispering, if you have not heard me speaking, then I find myself obligated to scream so that you will listen to me and to yourself." It was then that an automobile accident occurred and my life flashed before my eyes, as in one of James Cameron's best films, and I knew I had reached a fork in the road where it was urgent to define the path I would take.

In 3D there are different emotional energies and thoughts that resonate in low spectrums of light, and when our vibrations descend into those spectrums, they penetrate us. That is how I found myself wrapped in envy, jealousy, and all the things a person driven by those emotions may be overwhelmed by. Fortunately, a wise woman, one of the many angels to have crossed my path, had programmed a pink quartz crystal for me because she said I had to protect myself from something very powerful that only Love could protect me from. After the accident, I followed her instructions. It was this same crystal that I'd seen shatter before my very eyes at the moment of the accident. As it broke into a thousand pieces, it seemed to be giving its life for mine. It is perhaps one of the biggest acts of love that I have ever experienced, and it was from that moment that my deafness toward the universe disappeared and I began the magical journey toward the Quantum leap of Universal Consciousness.

I remember well how those crystal beings spoke to me when I was a child; I was no longer afraid to listen to them, and I began the great adventure of contacting the speaker of one of those crystals personified into a female angel: Katrina Raphaell. After having read her trilogy and allowing each crystal that appeared to give me messages of healing and growth and more, I decided to travel to Kappa, Hawaii. This was a very Pleiadian place charged with Lemurian energy, as well. It was there that I was blessed with being able to receive from this extraordinary woman her most intimate secrets, aided by these crystal gods. I was able to "speak" with one impressive crystal that communicates the movements of the planets, and through which Lady Gaia's energy network expands to create great changes and healing. I also received what was the beginning of my collection of healing crystals, which to this day are still with me physically and spiritually. Those crystals have all of my respect and that of each of the people and beings that have come into contact with them.

After this experience, I began to venture into anything that had to do with healing, such as Universal Healing, Gold Light, Reiki, Pranic Healing, and different methods of meditation. I received a Master's Degree in Neurolinguistic Programming (NLP) and thus received important knowledge on the human being and its physical, mental, emotional, spiritual and energetic behavior in 3D.

I had not yet left my job as a successful executive, nor had I stopped practicing various professions such as design, photography, publicity, marketing, or architecture, due to fear of the lack of security that a stable job and income brings. Once again the universe had to raise its voice so that I could let go of this crutch that I knew was the antithesis of Love: fear paralyzes and Love is a motor; one darkens while the other brightens; the former makes us sick while the latter heals us. This, after all that I have lived, is no longer a theory but strong evidence. I have many stories about the transmutation of one into the other.

Today, I give infinite thanks to all those techniques of light, healing and love that came to my life, as they were the key that opened my senses, allowing me to recognize the true Being that exists in me, which is ultimately the same being that exists in us All.

I would like to share with you parts of a channeling that Kryon did for me in January 2012 through Marina Mecheva, another angel in my path who allowed the high vibration in me to be recognized and to act out its true mission:

[...] your soul integrates the colors of beauty in such a profound way that a lot of what you perceive as reality is esoteric, sensual, harmonious, and similar to the beauty of your soul. There is softness in you, a childlike innocence that you have not lost, even after so much time. You have come to this planet to sustain the ray of innocence of the inner child, the pattern of joy in the terrestrial plane [...]

[...] the mystic part of the universe that you belong to, for you are a part of the creation of the universe, is quite linked to the joy and innocence because, you see, the first among you that are the creators of these dimensional reality had to be capable of maintaining this joy, the highest levels of it, so as to allow creation to flow through your breath, through your laugh, through the song of creation as you move further into these realities [...]

[...] there is so much knowledge within you, such a power within you, within the innocence of that child [...] You are so capable of communicating with the highest of vibrations without being spiritual because you will see it is a gift that you come with, a breath for life that is unique, different from the rest [...]

[...] your way of seeing this world is quite different from the way others see it [...]

[...] There are such beautiful colors in your energy field [...] the beauty in your soul is like a bouquet of spring flowers that spread their lovely scent everywhere, a color so radiant it can be seen from the other side; the colors are the following; a bright and radiant violet that is almost indigo, bright radiant blue, yellow, pink, and red, all combined in a ray of elemental energy that projects itself through you in everything you do. You spread this special light into all of your dimensional experience [...] the Indigo Ray is part of your predominant expression, regardless of the time you were born into your human body, because you express the characteristics of a new human being anyway [...]

[...] When you came to this planet you were not ready for this human experience, and thus the colors in your field were closer to the violet ray, but now, through the strengthening of your conviction, in your understanding of how the world must change, you explore this Indigo Ray with great courage as you remember why you came to this planet.

[...] you came closer to these dimensions like a wave of energy [...] to experience a different vibrational frequency, a different dimension to see the beauty in which your light manifests [...]

[...]That is how you, like a wave of original energy, manifested through the Indigo-Violet Ray, approached the planet [...] pieces within you decided to be a part of this experience and while you approached earth you felt for the first time what it feels like to vibrate so low, so as to be able to be a part of this physicality. This body is very new for you, breathing is new; in fact if we described you, we would not even call you human; there is a specific name for your race in the universe, part of it being the name for which you are known, another part a sound that activates a greater understanding of who you are, because in reality a human language will not be able to tell you where you come from [...]

Not even your scientists or astronomers know the existence of the system from which you come; it is very similar to the Pleiadian system, the 'seven sisters,' but different, much more profound in expression; it contains rays from Source in the manner that it expresses the original light, abundance, and beauty [...]

You can, starting today, not even speak of spiritual things and you will still be more spiritual than many of the human beings who are just waking up, simply because you are there to be exactly that: light. Light from the Indigo Ray that is there to change society's old status quo, which is there to create integrity and truth, which is there to show people the truth, regardless of where you are, to show them what is right, because you carry an innate understanding of what must be done, of what systems must be implemented so that humanity can finally begin to understand energy the way you understand it in the place you come from. [...]

[...] How you choose to implement this ray of original energy is in your hands [...] in order to be closer to the universal light systems, human law must become universal law [...]

[...] a being of such high vibrational frequency can only lower one to two percent of its soul to be able to go into a three-dimensional body. Therefore most of your being is still in the space that you remember in your deepest of dreams, a cosmic dream that exists in the heartbeat of the universe [...]

[...] there is a legion of energies in the invisible world that will always be a part of you [...]

[...] your field has the opportunity to create richness, abundance, anchorage; you are learning to express energy in form and the process is quite beautiful to watch [...]

[...] you, specifically, can build the attributes of a new energy, of a developing world; new ideas, new concepts, original executions; you are so unique in all that you believe because this Indigo Ray in your field needs this, calls for it [...] You will create such a powerful magnet for the world, that you will completely change the current perspective of things [...] it's a very powerful energy, a hook, to be able to move things; energy is movement, and the way you create movement is through inspiration, novelty, good practices, new activities, new things [...] part of your role in coming to the planet is to create new structures, new atmospheres, new businesses, new ways of doing politics, medicine, new forms of everything [...] if you continue with your conviction there is no way you will not be able to create a better society [...]

[...] you will establish the base of this in the new year, this year will be quite beneficial for you because you will let go of many old ways of thinking, you will break the status quo, you will let go of old models of thought and you allow new inspiration to create everything to be able to change what must be changed so that you may create the movement that will speed things up and bring money to everyone.

[...] your reality is the heart that builds the world [...] so celebrate the beginning of this year; expect the unexpected and create the promise [...]

And so it is!

Many months went by before I could digest this powerful information. I had to travel far from my country and my close family, on my own, hoping to find my cosmic family and dive into Layer Eight of my DNA. There I could remember part of the beginning of this existence, where art inspired every one of my senses, and the wind, ocean, and soft touch of Barcelona's sun would help me remember that I am not alone. There is a legion of incarnate and disincarnate light beings who are here as part of the team working on getting this message to millions of people to be able to build this desired Earth, free of ego, crystal clear, and transparent.

Just as you read it, dear reader, I fervently believe in a **New Earth** and that 2012 was not the year the world would end. The fact that you are reading this means you are living proof; what ended in 2012 were the old structures, the civilization of powers as things stood then. In 2012, dramatic change began.*

For years there has been talk of a global conspiracy. Many people believe there's a global agenda that has been carried out for many generations, involving premeditated events by certain people and organizations. Supporters of this theory affirm that the majority of human beings are asleep and have not awakened to their true divine nature, due to the strategies of a powerful elite that keeps us distracted, feeding our sense of fear so that we are always synced with lower frequencies. It is also said that through many mechanisms they have managed to induce us to compete against each other, dismissing the idea of unity, and thus distancing ourselves from our true inner power. This theory says that they do not want us to wake up but to continue to be dominated, enslaved by a system created by them.

This powerful elite is associated with the use of techniques such as brain-washing, media manipulation, fumigation of the population with chemtrails, the generation of earthquakes and seaquakes with machines of unknown technologies, the creation of impure vaccines and viruses to make humanity sick, the creation of economic crises and political parties whose bottom line is to keep us divided, the manipulation of world organizations, and other achievements that coincide with the actual reality of the planet. If you would like more information on this topic, you can look into any of David Icke's books; he has been a tireless seeker of this type of evidence and has brought to light the actions of this global conspiracy.

The question is not whether these powerful groups exist, or whether everything attributed to them is true, or even the veracity of the global conspiracy theory; what is important is to understand that all this has lead us to operate from fear, and the resulting frequency that is tuned into our bodies and minds in the frequency of illness, lack, competition, separation, cowardice, poverty, and limitation. Fear is naturally in our brains, since the mechanism of thought brings us to a series of hypotheses on future events; and a hypothesis is nothing more than a supposition that may or may not happen in a future that does not exist and that we only imagine in the only possible reality: the present.

My Beginning

Our dear poet Facundo Cabral used to say that we follow the future our whole lives, and that when it arrives, it becomes the present; that is to say, it no longer exists. Therefore, we are consumed by an illusion of something that is not real and, besides not being real, it pushes us away from our true nature, in which we're one hundred percent responsible for what we think, feel, say and do in regard to what we desire in our lives, instead of giving free rein to that which we do not want and become paralyzed believing in illusion. We are unhappy before it even arrives because we believe it to be true and thus end up manifesting the closest reality.

So, how do we change that frequency of fear? By activating within us the frequency of Love, which cannot be achieved with the mind, but only from the heart. Since we have lived in the frequency or vibration of fear for eons, it is necessary to not only heal the memories of this lifetime but also all our other manifestations of life, and something even more potent: the memories of all the civilizations and galaxies that vibrate and have vibrated in the frequency derived from fear. To achieve this, we must start from the beginning, with the Earth. Our beloved light-Earth planet vibrates at the frequency of the Indigo Ray and it is now necessary for it to anchor itself to the DNA of all its inhabitants to vibrate at the frequency of the only thing that is real, which is Love.

You, dear reader, belong to this movement. The movement of Freedom: freedom of expression, art, science and spirituality. This creates divine perfection with each thought, word, emotion and action where Unity is responsible. You are part of this transformation. You are the protagonist of the new Earth, of the new Jerusalem. The universe has put this book in your hands because it knows that you are ready to receive this information at this time. Prepare to leap, or rather to fly, without boundaries into time and space, into quantum reality, where everything that resonates from Love is possible.

* In order to be able to create said change, it is important to manifest it not only theoretically but in reality as well, thus the importance of syncing ourselves to the same energy on a daily basis. This is why we have designed a series of seminars and workshops in which this powerful tool imprints itself in our being and teaches us not as a "healing technique" but as a way of life, a tool to aid in any activity that occurs in daily life. Amplify the information found in the seminars by watching this video: **Seminar:** http://bit.ly/1glsWJ1

For more gifts and experiences from IRB: Transforming Fear Into Love, go to:
bit.ly/XimenaDuqueValencia_IRB

I want to subscribe and receive my free gift:
bit.ly/IRB_PeaceMeditation

PART ONE

The End of the Old

Chapter 1
2012: Transitioning to the New Galactic Dawn

It's about a new path where one builds oneself.
I found this path to be common in many cultures.
From the most remote ancient times, different schools of thought
covertly taught the only possible freedom for man: his voluntary transformation.

René Rebetez

Many people speak of Mayan prophecies and the date announced on their calendar as the end of our civilization. To speak of the prophecy is to speak of prediction and whenever we predict, a manifestation of thought is materialized; therefore, these types of prophecies become apocalyptic and inevitable. But we must remember that the future does not exist; it is only a projection of our thoughts. The power of emotion empowers our thoughts, which are reinforced and regulated by words and especially the power of the verb; thus, action is coherent with manifestation. In this way, we create the future each day with the only thing we have: the present moment and our consciousness. Therefore, I believe that the Mayans left us a wise guide for preparing ourselves for planetary events.

Thanks to current events and the current evolution, along with the guidance that helps us break old paradigms, we can create great change, great transitions. It is the endless changes in customs, ideas, beliefs, culture and technical knowledge, that characterize us as the true human race, in constant evolution, developing a new perspective in areas such as economics, politics, culture, religion and science, where the discovery of true wellness will be found.

The human race has experienced many "ends" of the world such as the Great Flood, yet we still inhabit the planet. The descension that we have witnessed, which began to change in 2013, is one of materialism and division, of limits and fear, the way we have identified ourselves for so long, and the reason we have killed and disrespected each other over the course of our diverse history. This time is the end of death as we know it and the birth of the extraordinary. We must feel blessed to be in this moment that, beyond the chaos that fear wishes to instill within us, is the opportunity to create common wellbeing with richness, abundance, the sacred, and All of Us being One.

This is not a moment but a transition that begins inside each of us, in the center of our hearts, where the frequency of Love is found and where we may reflect, radiate and multiply the best of ourselves without selfishness, from Oneness, from a point of sharing and bonding, from the deepest, most complete and sacred part of ourselves.

Just as the Earth has four seasons in the year that change every three months, the galaxy too has these seasons that occur every 26,000 years. The date predicted by the Mayans, the 21st of December, 2012, was the beginning of the galactic Spring, just as Spring begins on Earth on March 21 in the Northern Hemisphere and the 21st of September in the Southern hemisphere; this doesn't happen in a moment but is a three-month-long transition. The following day, the 22nd, we do not see blossoms on trees but only snow melting and, some weeks later, the trees showing their first leaf buds; later still, flowers bloom; and, a month or month and a half later, we witness their full bloom. It is the same situation cosmically. The new galactic dawn allows us to melt the snow in our hearts, feel the cold and dark fade away, then later enjoy the buds beginning to appear; for now, we are only at the beginning of the process.

Let us then not expect immediate blossoming. Let us live with utmost confidence in the perfect process of the blossoming of the great light, and let us persist through joy, acceptance and the ability to endure the pain that must accompany the magic of transformation. Let's begin removing each layer that protects us from the cold, as they are no longer necessary. Let us continue baggage-free, free from attachments and beliefs, free to experience this great transformation that IRB proposes. The key is the light, the light that gives life to Love: The *Living Light*.

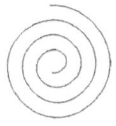

Chapter II

The Key is the Light

Emotion is the chief source of all becoming conscious.
There can be no transforming of darkness into light nor apathy into movement without emotion.

Carl Jung

Throughout the history of humanity, various civilizations have worshiped the Sun as a god and erected great monuments to honor him, including some of the pyramids in Mexico and Egypt. We have, as "civilized beings," stopped worshipping the great sun king and only commune with it to warm ourselves or to tan; we only miss the sun on occasion, when it is hiding behind clouds. For the rest, we are so used to its morning routine that we forget the sun's importance and vitality. It is not about going back to worshipping the sun, but of connecting to its light to anchor it within our being and to be able to illuminate our entire world exactly as it does.

Physically and astrologically speaking, the past few years have been marked by what scientists call solar storms. We have been told that these explosions are occurring more and more frequently and that we have been affected by them in the past, such as in the Carrington Event of 1859, which managed to disrupt the then poorly developed communication systems in both North America and Europe. The Carrington Event had no drastic consequences because the technology of our civilization was still in its beginnings; if it occurred today, our artificial satellites would cease to work, causing interrupted radio signals, and there would be electrical blackouts of continental proportions, interrupting electrical service for weeks.

None of this is to scare anyone or cause panic or allow the frequencies of fear to once again take us over. It's important that we are aware that without electricity we would have no power in our homes, as most of our appliances depend on it. In our cities, the failure of gas stations, traffic lights, stores, automatic teller machines, super markets and countless other commodities, would also result in chaos. Banks would not be able to verify the amounts in our accounts because everything is stored in computers that require electricity. If something similar to the Carrington Event were to happen today, according to the National Academy of Sciences of the United States, the electric network of the country, and thus the rest of the world, would be vulnerable, satellites would no longer orbit, cell phones would cease to work, as would global positioning systems (GPS), control towers that commercial flights depend on, and so on, with countless elements that we depend on every day. So, would we believe that it was the end of the world? Or, better, the beginning of a new era?

Only when we understand that we don't need external things in order to live, will we begin to discover the power that we have within, which we currently are not using. We have the power to create with all living beings new systems based in harmony, balance and love. We can sync ourselves to the frequencies of chaos, or we can prepare for the transition. Activating the interior Sun, connecting to the Living Light, these things allow us to recognize our origin, awakening Source.

Chapter III

Awakening

Creativity is inventing, experimenting, growing, taking risks, breaking rules, making mistakes… and having fun.

Mary Lou Cook

Awakening is an internal process, a change in human consciousness, and pure evolution. Evolution is Quantum in nature, which means non-linear, not just going forward; we can also talk about going back, back to the beginning, back to the memory of who we truly are, back to the Source of life where Living Light comes from. It is there that Quantum Physics allow us to understand that everything flows simultaneously, that everything is part of the same Whole.

Awareness is re-learning, going beyond what I first understood the day of my accident, knowing that we are in a place where we have chosen to live for much more reason than just being born, growing up, reproducing and dying. We have a mission in each of our existences, and that mission is always to evolve, and at the same time to serve others on their paths of evolution, to serve from love. And to be able to do that we each have a unique talent that is necessary to put in service to others.

To serve is the fundamental instrument of Love. It is very important to know exactly what serving consists of, quite apart from servility or sacrifice; many times we dedicate our lives to serving the underprivileged, then we feel a need to create more disadvantaged people in order to fulfill our calling. To be of service is to discover our innate talent and to make it our ultimate goal to share our creativity with others, keeping our minds and spirits open to receive just compensation for this contribution.

In that vein, awakening individually is important, but we tend to stay in that individualism; to foment separation is to halt evolution. The work we collectively do is priority, since Lady Gaia must also awake and ascend to superior or lighter densities. The consciousness of the human being changes constantly, since it is the perspective from which we see things happening; as we evolve, our perspective widens, and it is essential to evolve to higher levels until we have made that quantum leap, the ascension that occurs every 26,000 years, which, according to Mayan prophecies, recurred in December of 2012.

Eckhart Tolle talks to us about old structures collapsing; that is what we must be prepared for, to build the new Earth from the heart, from the Love that can only be found in energy that is balanced and harmonious. We can destroy ourselves, along with this world, through individuality, division and fear — or be born again in a world based on togetherness and Love. True power is within each of us; this has been said by many, and understanding this is the first step in understanding that we are all the creators of our own realities. We can continue to create discord from our spiritual slumber, or we can create a reality based on love and founded on the awareness of being awake. Many have said this before… why, then, is the long-awaited magical awakening taking so long?

Because, though we talk about it, our belief system attached to these old unstable structures keeps us from making the final leap and confronting our own belief systems; it's a very difficult process of acceptance. To see the old belief structures of someone else coming down can be distressing, but seeing our own belief system fail scares us more, and fear keeps us from loving. That is why this book was born, that is why IRB is happening, not only to knock down the old structures that keep us in a world that is asleep — a world full of veils and cobwebs that blind us to the existence of our true selves — but also to try, through individual healing, to heal our collective history, the DNA of our people and our nations; it is to awaken consciousness for a complete change on the Earth.

Every movement and manifestation that has happened up until this moment to help us understand the old government and institutional models are not compatible with the new energy, which has opened our consciousness to change, and it's time for that change to manifest into physical reality. That is the fundamental purpose of INDIGO RAY BALANCING (IRB): to be the protagonists of the new Earth, for us to sync with the transparency, the clarity of the Koradi race, the new race that populates the Earth, with all the information in the spectrum of the Indigo Ray that allows us to Be One, respecting the richness of diversity, allowing us to build a new society that gives priority to life over monetary or political interests; we will only achieve this when we release old paradigms from within each of ourselves and from our personal DNA.

How would you like to be able to communicate, not by internet but by a telepathic net? What if, instead of paying airline tickets, you could simply go anywhere through teleportation? What if you could be in many places at once? What if you no longer needed to spend a fortune on doctors, hospitals and medicine because you could simply use your gifts of healing? What if your communications were no longer limited because you do not speak through words but through the Living Light of the heart that connects you to the DNA network where we are All One? What if all this were a reality that we could build with a change from the depths of our belief systems? If you want the answer to these questions to be yes and for it to become a reality, then you are ready to wake up, accessing the totality of the information that is offered by IRB.

The universal law of free will is what allows us to choose. THIS IS THE TIME to choose wisely, from the heart, where we want to go and what we want to do. It is up to us to make into a reality the Golden Era that began in the end of 2012, consolidated in 2013, and comes to a definite anchoring around 2018, to materialize the universal balance from the Indigo Ray which allows us to sync as One with the center of our galaxy and to recognize the potential of Love, which can transform fear.

> TO THINK DIFFERENTLY IS TO CREATE DIFFERENT REALITIES.

Elevating our frequencies when we wake up allows us to sync with our Spiritual Source, recognized by its true laws, not the laws that consume us in our human limits but the laws that maximize the unlimited being within our sacred Being.

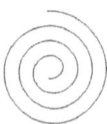

Chapter IV

The Master Key

You must be careful never to allow doubt to paralyze you. Always make the decisions you need to make, even if you're not sure you're doing the right thing.

Paulo Coelho

One of the universal laws expressed by Hermes Trismegisto in his book The Kybalion, tells us that everything is mind. That means thought is the beginning of creation. Many belief systems in the areas of philosophy and religion are based on fear and sin. Sentences such as, "If you do this or that, God will punish you," were imbedded over centuries into the collective consciousness through faulty religious teachings. With the passing of the years and the evolution of higher religions that are the pillar of humanity, the narrative of a Punishing God has finally been replaced by that of a Loving God.

Pope John Paul II, the supreme minister of the Catholic Church between 1978 and 2005, expressed on July 28, 2003, two days before dying, "Hell exists, but we do not know who's there." A week before that statement, he had talked about Heaven. In both cases, the saintly father affirmed that neither Heaven nor Hell were physical places. In the case of Hell, he insisted that:

The images of hell that Sacred Scripture presents to us must be correctly interpreted. They show the complete frustration and emptiness of life without God. Rather than a place, hell indicates the state of those who freely and definitively separate themselves from God, the source of all life and joy. [...]

"Eternal damnation," therefore, is not attributed to God's initiative because in his merciful love he can only desire the salvation of the beings he created. In reality, it is the creature that closes himself to His love. Damnation consists precisely in definitive separation from God, freely chosen by the human person and confirmed with death that seals his choice forever. [...]

This means that Hell is an idea that was invented and sustained for centuries so that humans would do no harm for fear of punishment, and when we sync ourselves to the frequencies of fear, our thoughts, which are the master key, immediately open the door to hell, making us live in dissonance, unbalanced, in violence, limitation and illusion; we identify with form, poverty, illness, anger, rancor, and all that is worthy of an infernal state.

In the same way, our thoughts allow us to open the door to Heaven, the state found in communion with Joy, which is the personification of pure Love, allowing us to live in a state of co-creation, balance, harmony, and awareness of our eternal present. This is where true power is found, within the definitive connection to our primary source found in the heaven that is in our DNA, not in the power of manipulation provoking the sense of separation from Source. It is in separation that we believe God is found outside ourselves and that we must implore him to turn his merciful gaze toward us and throughout our prayers concede us a place in Heaven.

Only when we truly understand that Heaven is within us, that we are all sacred, that God is not a separate being but a level of consciousness existing in our DNA, the source of all that is, will we be able to connect our totality to the concept of unity in Love. Not unity with the material which separates us, but from Spirit, which is the origin of body and mind as incarnate spiritual beings in this density to experience ourselves as humans, as the universe's project that is evolving toward that which is truly sacred.

Our world as we know it pushes us to compete and to be separate from others from the day we are born. We are divided by race, religion, social status and class, in possessing and not possessing, in being better or worse, and each group believes they own the truth, to the point of starting wars and murdering to defend that truth. All this chaos has been created by the ignorance of not knowing ourselves as spiritual beings, since we Are All One and possess the same infinite power within ourselves, in our nucleus, in our cells, where we are all identical though with different missions. Each of us together make up the totality.

Why have "the powers that be" hidden this knowledge? Because if we wake up to this reality, the few that believe they hold power would cease to wield it over the rest of us, and that, in this world of illusion where we have existed for so long, would mean the end of manipulation, the end of the few who control the banking system, the political system, transnational corporations, pharmaceutical companies, and the mass communication media and more.

We are on this planet at the level of 3D consciousness living a role in a game; the problem is that we were not given clear rules and we are playing blindfolded. The blindfold is the conjunction of our five earthly senses. Our work has been to discover these rules of the game and remove the blindfold, developing our senses beyond the physical, communicating at more expanded levels within ourselves and going beyond the confinement of the limiting mind-body ribbon of perception in which most humans finds themselves, because the system was designed to keep us there without any maneuverability.

Those of us abandoning the confines of the body are doing so because we have been able to open ourselves to a higher level of consciousness. This doesn't mean that we are special, or Messianic, it just means we have decided to open our minds to another level of perception and knowledge and to change our point of view in regard to what we see, hear, or feel with our five senses to recognize our divine essence. We can all achieve this.

The important part of all this is to understand, as David Icke said, "One man cannot change the world. But one man can communicate the message that can change the world!" So this is a key factor; it is not about the individual but the information that has transformative power. It's as if our DNA had software installed to limit its true divine extension. Why is this software installed? Because we only manipulate that which we think is stronger than us. Meaning, we are yielding our true power to beings that are extraordinarily limited compared to human potential; that's why they must use humanity and keep us from awakening, since that would mean "game over."

Without paying attention to what type of religion we belong to or the type of philosophy we share, it is necessary to awaken. For this, we must access the quantum language that allows us to communicate with our DNA to access our true creative potential, expanding our consciousness beyond the five senses.

Our genetic code is of divine origin, but external greed has blocked our super-consciousness and true power, just as J.J. Hurtak indicated in his book, The Keys of Enoch, the true book of knowledge. This truth has been kept hidden, perpetuated in secret in coded form under the symbol of the Holy Grail.

Itzen Caan who has been researching and decoding Mayan and Atlantean symbols for over twenty years, tells us in her writing, Memories of Atlantis:

> [...] to maintain power and control over the masses, this knowledge became a forbidden topic, and to talk about it would alarm those who, by their own decree, allotted themselves the power and dominion of humans, immediately

executing imperious actions as punishment for those that spoke of anything having to do with issues such as, for example, that descended gods united with earthly women leaving their solar-cosmic genetic inheritance.

Part of the manipulation found in religious dogmas have pushed us away from profound truths such as the study of sacred science, ancient knowledge, metaphysics, the human essence, and even alchemical nature, by labeling anything that touched upon profound truths as "Satanism," "profane," "condemned" and "witchcraft," placing those same labels on anything having to do with the study or discovery of our original and essential nature, or the awakening and opening of consciousness. The most frustrating part of this fraud put together by the manipulative elite lies in the alienation of the woman with anything having to do with profound knowledge and anything that leads to awakening. There is deep fear of the development of her natural power, since it is the feminine aspect in both women and men that activates the sixth sense, or intuition, that connects us to our true being. It is the master key that opens the door to the truth and the discovery that our feminine essence represents the Grail as an ancestral and historical truth, not a mythical one.

This also means that the true power of sexual energy has been mutilated, denigrating not only sex itself, but woman as well, since discovering our true and original essence lies in sexual intercourse, and through this high-level union of the cosmic-spiritual, we give leeway to the maximum power of creation that we humans possess.

To further keep us from the power of feminine essence, the symbolism of the prostitute was presented, combined with the history of Mary Magdalene which directly condemned any woman that came close to the ancient wisdom and Christic knowledge, thereby preventing the unveiling of this historical lie.

Both educational and religious dogmas have blocked the path to the truth, suffocating our intuition through mandates such as, "don't ask, but just believe everything we tell you." And if you try to think differently, or get close to the truth, then you are threatened with condemnation of the soul, if you speak, believe, or practice anything different from these dogmas, and even more so if you try to investigate or clarify the information given. Enormous walls have been erected to blind us from the truth, erected from norms, sins, demons and fears that have submerged humanity into obscurity and blindness, forcing it to need crutches to be able to live, generating codependency, separation and veiled slavery.

WHEN LIGHT COMES, DARKNESS DISAPPIERS

This plan of manipulation has attempted to nullify feminine energy, distorting womankind and sexual energy to gain power and control over mankind, driving it onto lower planes and completely distorting its protagonistic role through lies and fear. Light and darkness simply indicate the existence of these two polarities in the world from source; the polarity of light reflecting truth, and darkness reflecting fear and lies. One way or another, though it may seem paradoxical, each has a part in evolution, but if we choose one and fight against the other, we become separate and succumb to the lie and forget who we truly are, generating chaos and significantly slowing down our transition.

When we succumb to the polarity of fear, we give power to manipulation and allow the oppression and enslavement of humanity. It is only from this knowledge, from Point Zero, that we can transcend the limits and co-create a reality of balance and harmony for all. Polarity leads us to duality and separates us from Oneness.

The imposition of masculine energy in the world and the discrimination against feminine energy, moved by the desire to obtain individual power and selfish personal growth, was what caused the imbalance that still reigns on Earth. The unity of philosophy and the metaphysical, the visible and the invisible, of opposites, is what allows us to merge the duality at high spiritual levels, balancing the polar energies and permitting the balance and harmony of the whole being and the world.

There was a climactic moment in history in which all important feminine icons were eliminated; historical, ancient, mythological and religious. Any evidence of their participation in teaching, life guiding, and defending positive life values, was eliminated. There was a time when women had the same leadership weight, perhaps even more so, in religious and political decisions, to the point of maintaining mankind in a golden era of harmony and equality in both polar forces: masculine and feminine. In the book of Genesis, the Bible says balance was disrupted by members of the priesthood when they distorted the original truth, preaching that woman, by "listening to the snake" and eating the prohibited fruit, caused divine wrath with her disobedience and sin, thus expelling man and woman from paradise and condemning humankind to suffering. This resulted in a great symbolic turn of events and a hidden agenda of guilt and contempt toward womankind.

This manipulation was brought on by the religious elite who wished to undermine the extrasensory perception and intuition of woman. The symbolism of listening to the snake and its consequential access to knowledge and Wisdom (eating the apple, the forbidden fruit) is no different from having access to the Divine Universal mind, represented by the tree of knowledge. It is due to this natural feminine characteristic that in ancient times, there were women called Pythonesses, (which comes from the term python, or great snake, meaning great knowledge) who were women who dedicated themselves to cultivating their intuitive gift and maintained their mental-spiritual connection through the natural access of original Divine Wisdom.

The symbolism shows us that woman, not man, through her intuition and spiritual connection, can hear and understand the language of the serpent in the tree of science, of good and evil. This means that it is the feminine polarity that possesses the innate sensibility and perception that connects the ethereal-spiritual plane where true knowledge resides, to manifest it later in the physical plane through the masculine energy represented in man. The snake is nothing more than a representation of the sapience or natural Wisdom, taken as a direct fruit, the apple of the great tree, the ceiba tree of the Mayans, the divine energy that enlivens the entire universe. Both the feminine and masculine polarities are intrinsic to man and woman, not mere characteristics of him or her, the erroneous belief imprinted to override the innate connection to Wisdom that flows within the information of the quantum field.

Feminine polarity, represented by Eve, has the gift of intuition and sensibility, of the pythoness, capable of obtaining the ether, the divine essence or Wisdom, through the symbol of the apple, which represents the master or divine mind. Through it she shares it with Adam, the masculine polarity, symbol of intelligence and great strength, thereby creating together the wonders that gave life to great civilizations in ancient golden ages. By distorting this sacred knowledge, by enforcing this lie and integrating it into a plan of manipulation, feminine polarity — which balances the duality of the world — was misrepresented to block out sensitivity, subtle perception, what is referred to as the sixth sense, as well as love and maternal energy, which is nothing less than the maximum power of creation, the key characteristic of this complementary energy.

As we have said, this did not happen only in women, a the feminine polarity, essence or energy, is also found in men. We see it as his more sensitive side. Hence the gradual dulling of the capacity to connect spiritually to the direct access to Wisdom and the understanding of the non-separateness, of the absolute oneness with the cosmos. The idea of separation disconnected humanity from its own nature, from its surroundings, from Mother Nature, from the energetic balance, and has made us forget that in essence we are pure Consciousness.

The opening of consciousness that leads us to once again find balance, and the consequent elevation of our vibrational level, gives us expedited access to the multidimensional. The Living Light that creates the essence of love with its predominantly feminine energy, in perfect balance with the masculine energy, is the only thing capable of returning the world and the human race to perfect harmony. This cosmic, subtle, feminine energy, the bringer of Love, comes through IRB, and not to impose itself but to unify duality, awakening the integral and unique human spirituality, the connection to nature, and the launching of metaphysical capacities. This is our essence, and divine genetic cosmic composition that connects us in a direct and powerful way to the quintessential creative essence, and it is the pure heritage of our real and true origin.

> ONLY WHEN COMPLETELY UNITED ARE WE THE PERFECT EXPRESSION OF CREATION.

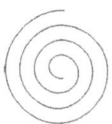

Chapter V

Evolution

*Taking initiative does not mean being pushy, obnoxious or aggressive.
It does mean recognizing our responsibility
to make things happen.*

Stephen Covey

Have you ever felt that life is unfair? We see children starving and dying of thirst while others waste the bounty they are blessed with. And what about children who needlessly die or are victims of violence? All those kids suffer physical or health issues from birth while others enjoy good health, safety, comfort and everything else deemed important to well-being!

Who has the power to decide whether we are born into a good family in a country without war, in a home without lack — or seriously ill in a nation wracked by violence? Why is it that so many beings do nothing but suffer throughout their lives, while others enjoy a life of peace and harmony in their surroundings?

Many superficial answers can be found if one asks a scientist, a priest, or a person in a state of unconsciousness. This was the situation I found myself in when I began to ask these types of questions. Is it simply about luck, or is there divine will?

In truth, nothing in this universe is determined by chance, and we come to the understanding, after a long time of evolving our religious philosophies, that what is referred to as God is Love, not punishment. Therefore, the two superficial answers given above are, in my view, null and void. Einstein once said, "God does not play dice with the universe."

Throughout this journey, I have found people completely attached to their low vibrations who blame others for everything that happens to them, believing their suffering is caused by curses, spells, and dark forces. But is there such a thing as blame? My answer is a resounding no! Yes, there exists responsibility for our actions, which are in turn fostered by our emotions and thoughts. Some results are immediate, while others gestate and bear fruit after a while, perhaps even after several incarnations. Just as a bean sprouts in a much shorter time than an apple, likewise our actions gestate in time and space, especially in this 3D world in which we live to experience, learn and evolve.

Responsibility allows us to analyze elements that have participated in our actions, to be able to choose with Wisdom whether we want to repeat them or to obtain a different result. When we change our actions from a place of responsibility, we allow ourselves to learn from experience, generating evolution.

By co-creating the events and conditions in our life, we affect the life of everything that surrounds us. This means that, not only are we responsible for the results in our lives, but we also influence the results of others. So, are we responsible for what happens to others? My answer is once again a resounding no! People who share their lives with us are, in turn, responsible for their own co-creations, and just as sickness, poverty, abuse, and violence have been lessons of choice, those who facilitate them have been our most powerful teachers. In turn, we have been chosen to teach others, as in one big soul family. We Are All One.

When we anchor this energy of responsibility, we effect change in our universe and our immediate surroundings. The most harmonious way to achieve this is by allowing ourselves to practice the most powerful lesson that our teacher Jesus left us during his incarnation on Earth: Love thy neighbor as thyself. (Read that closely: as thyself.)

Are you aware of how you love yourself? Because one can only give what one has and can only reflect what we think we are, I invite you to refine the idea you have of yourself so that the image you are projecting can be linked to your essence in its true divine and spiritual density.

We are spiritual beings living a human experience. We are energy manifested in a material world. Earth is the great university that allows us to create our own experiences to foster evolution. The new energy gives us the option to bypass what for so many centuries was known as karma. Evolution helps us understand that what we used to view as problems and challenges are really teachers and friends that lead us to relinquish overt control, and we understand from our divine essence that we create problems in our reality so that we can become masters, not to succumb to them, nor to feel guilt generated from a state of unconsciousness.

Conscious acceptance of everything as part of a divine plan, and acceptance of the perfection of the present moment — the only thing that is real — removes from of our minds the need to label every situation. We must stop labeling and simply accept things as they are, without the judgment or condemnation that empowers harmful or euphoric emotions that can only create an ego-based reality; the ego only wishes to manipulate and judge, empowered by the fear caused by attachment. The big secret is to consciously learn from our experiences and move on.

Karma was the greatest teacher of pain and suffering. THIS IS THE TIME to learn from another teacher: Consciousness. Before coming into this human existence on Earth, our energy, our souls, choose the circumstances we wish to experience in order to learn and continue to evolve. When we are born, we come to this side of the veil where we get lost in the illusion we can call "the image in the mirror;" it appears to be real, but it's only the reflection of the reality we create each moment, a hologram of who we are personifying.

The veil is sometimes so thick that we forget the choices we made or why we made them. In this state, attachment and suffering create separation from our essence and this leads to illness, unbalanced relationships and the engulfing belief that "the fall" is a reality. We must tear away the veil and recognize our divine essence in order to embrace the totality of our magnificence and stop trying to correct the image in the mirror.

What we have called God for so many years, never forgets us and never punishes us. God is not a separate entity from us; it is all that exists, and all that exists is God. God is DNA, it is Everything, it is Love, it is the only thing that is real. Therefore, we all evolve toward that inscrutable realization that everything is Love and Living Light. When that which is sacred radiates from our center, when we recognize God in all that Is, consciousness allows us to create a new reality from Love, from Abundance, from the perfection of all that Is, and we can honor every single manifestation of life from our absolute Oneness.

THIS IS THE TIME to awaken and escape the manipulation perpetrated by religious organizations, governments and powerful cabals that still cloud our consciousness, thus separating us from our divinity and creating a God we must fear. We must stop worshipping the senses that keep us in ignorance, completely halting our evolution toward a stable and balanced reality. Since December 2012, the evolution of the human race has been transforming the 3D along with the Earth, our beloved planet Gaia. This powerful university raises the vibration to the highest frequencies ever experienced, evolving to new unlimited dimensions. If you are reading this book, you have decided to be present at this crucial moment in human history as a protagonist of this great quantum leap. So enjoy the change of consciousness, and allow me to honor you, because only the bravest angels from the highest spheres have made the decision to evolve in these moments as vassals of light incarnate and as an example to the rest of humanity. It is a privilege and an honor to share these moments with you. Namaste!

The evolution that is allowing this era of change is allowing us to focus on our missions in life, our purpose, such as the election of our mastery, which I will discuss later. We are creating from divine consciousness a new reality with Love, to generate peace, harmony and perfect universal balance.

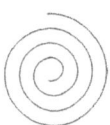

Chapter VI

Inter-dimensionality

Perhaps the greatest challenge of mankind at the dawn of the third millennium is understanding that we are not alone, that we share the universe. We find ourselves in the most beautiful adventure ever lived: the great luck of reuniting, celebrating, laughing and materializing from our own individuality a universe of collaboration among beings who, governed from an inner universe, live the dream of being universal Love.

Facundo Cabral

It is absolutely fascinating to be imbued with the order of the universe. The universe is All. When I saw the movie Contact (a 1997 adaptation of the science fiction novel Contact, written by Carl Sagan) I realized that I was not the only one who believes we are not alone but, compared to the millions of universes that exist out there, but a speck; we cannot, therefore, be so arrogant as to believe that we are alone, much less separate from the rest. As astronomer Ellie Arroway says in the movie, "If it is just us, seems like an awful waste of space."

In our Milky Way Galaxy alone, there are millions of planets, and as if that were not enough, in the universe exist millions and millions of galaxies, each with its respective millions of planets. Further, there is not one single universe but an infinite number of universes.

Our governments, our research agencies such as NASA, and even the Vatican, admit the truth of this. Things are happening such as the naming of the Malaysian astrophysicist, Mazlan Othman, as Ambassador of Space by the UN's Office for Outer Space Affairs (UNOOSA). So we have an Earth representative for aliens! CNN has reported in a press conference that UFO's oversee nuclear bases and have even deactivated nuclear missiles. Larry King Live, one of the most watched programs in the US, recently dedicated an hour to showing videos and eye-witness testimonies of UFO sightings. NASA has made a press release stating that there are two billion planets that share similar conditions with the Earth. Doctor Richard B. Hoover, an astrobiologist at NASA, has found proof of alien life in a meteorite. Jose Gabriel Fuentes, the priest in charge of the Vatican observatory, has admitted that the existence of alien life on other planets is possible. Monsignor Corrado Balducci, a member of the Vatican Clergy, has stated that extraterrestrial beings definitely exist and that they are superior to us with regard to spirituality and technology. These are but a few examples. There are real videos on YouTube in which we can see UFO's flying over places such as Utah, New York, Moscow and a mosque in Jerusalem. Pope John XXIII has said, "How small God would be if, after having created this immense universe, he had only populated Earth! That is not the God that I know." We could write entire pages about the life that exists out there.

What if we now spoke of the worlds inside the human being? We will expand further on this in Chapter XIX.

Have you ever thought about the external and internal worlds we can observe in this dimension? About the stories, lives, characters, parallel worlds and different dimensions that we are experiencing simultaneously, right here and now? Inter-dimensionality is something that we have all experienced in one way or another. For example, at a very basic level of Inter-dimensionality, while you are reading or listening to this, your brain is focused on the series of words that form our language. At the same time, perhaps you are listening to an external sound: cars passing by, birds singing, a blaring television, the barking of a dog, a melody or perhaps just your breathing. All of these events are diverse dimensions in your consciousness and you can recognize them by simply drawing your attention to them. Attention is what makes us present. If we do not pay attention, we do not realize what is happening. In the same way, if you decide to pay attention only to exterior sounds, even if you stop noticing your breathing, , it still exists, whether or not you're conscious of it.

This is the most basic level of Inter-dimensionality. By simply looking deeper, we discover that our inner world has many dimensions and realms, most of which are usually inaccessible to us because we have been trained to focus solely on a limited part of our inner experiences. In order to experience these inner worlds of perception, it is necessary to alter brain activity, whether that be through techniques such as meditation, or simply by being conscious of our inner silence, of the Presence, of the here and now.

Inter-dimensionality is very difficult to explain to someone raised under the limiting beliefs of the 3D world. We are angels, we have always been angels, and we will always be angels. We are temporarily on this planet as physical third-dimensional forms, and that part of us is human. Not all of our intellect is with us here; only a small portion is earth-bound; the rest remains hidden, though connected and available. The rest of our "I" remains in some other place, but still within the totality of our DNA. Being in many places at the same time is one of the gifts that we possess as supreme beings. We simply need to be conscious of past and future to be able to travel there and activate some of our abilities and talents in other lifetimes. Everything is here and now.

Part of being multidimensional is being able to access other dimensions, being able to see with our physical eyes what is considered non-physical — perhaps something that is not part of this world but some other plane of existence or dimension. It's important to understand that this space between worlds or dimensions, is also within ourselves. It is necessary to understand that space separates the worlds or dimensions that are, above all, found inside. Therefore, it is our own energy that leads us to others, and our real work now happens in the heart of thousands of groups inhabiting the Earth. When I say "groups," I'm not talking about cults or religions or philosophies that create separation, but informal gatherings of men and women willing to ride this wave of peace. The era of hidden assemblies and great missionaries is gradually fading away. Our mission now is to plant the seeds of change throughout the Earth with the help of many channels and a multitude of conscious forms that emit a specific type of harmony and strongly project an energetic field that radiates from the heart, from the purest form of Love, out to unlimited distances.

There are no chosen ones. Each of us chooses and attracts the light that elevates our surroundings, gathering a small spiritual family whose transparency is proportionate to ours. It is not about creating spiritual families that lead to closed, intolerant, hierarchical groups. Aggrandizement of the human ego creates separation. When we understand multi-dimensionality, we understand Oneness and are able to plant true fraternity of spirit. The era of teachers and disciples, of missionaries and fanatics is behind us. When we work in unity, the whole world receives and the whole world gives, in full and complete consciousness of being a promulgator of that everlasting Presence.

This Earth is one huge laboratory where different strains of humanity rub shoulders without our even realizing it. When we elevate our vibration, we can access very high spheres along

Inter-dimensionality

with our brothers and sisters. This is how the human "elite" and governments cannot hide their existence for much longer. Up until now they have made us believe that our intuitive truths have all been an illusion, that the superior brothers and sisters from these higher spheres do not exist, or that we should fear their presence.

All of this is changing, and love is the force behind this transformation that allows us to navigate through these dimensions without fear of diversity or change, accepting instead the riches provided for us.

Just as there is life beyond the Earth, there life in the hollow (inner) Earth, and it is just as important. Everything is fullness, even emptiness, which is far more than we dream. That is why responsibility over our thoughts is so important, because it not only creates our reality but that of all life close to us in our atmosphere. It is not only chemical pollution that is contaminating us, but our thoughts as well. When we understand our connection to all that Is, we stop living selfishly, thinking that we are on this earth alone and that it was made exclusively for our enjoyment, that it belongs to us in its entirety. The truth is simply that everything we see, even that which we do not see, is meant to be shared. We are the tenants on this world, not the landlords, and we are intimately connected because there is no empty space. Truly empty space does not exist; everything is made of life, and everything evolves in one direction. But only when we empty ourselves and experience the lightness of, not possessing but of sharing, do we merge into the emptiness. Only then are we truly full. It is one more dichotomy that becomes unified opposites flowing with Totality.

There are many dimensions, and one of the tools that we have at our disposal to access these dimensions is the pineal gland. One of the great scholars and, in my opinion, the one who knows the most on the topic, is David Wilcock, who said that this is not simply a bean-shaped gland of the endocrine system responsible for producing dimethyltryptamine (DMT) but also the strongest hallucinogen known to this day, responsible for displaying images in a dream state. It is so potent that it can take our consciousness through time and various dimensions. Wilcock confirmed that in the state immediately before death, great levels of DMT are produced, which is how dying people can enter higher dimensions of consciousness, observing beings that do not physically live in this 3D plane. DMT induces spontaneous mystical states at birth, in a state of deep rest, and when disembodied, activating clairvoyance. The Pranic energy that flows through the pineal gland is our receptive antenna, catapulting us into the past and the future. In that tiny gland, our entire Akashic Records are found. Further on, we will clearly explain what IRB does in people's lives so as to describe in-depth the importance of this gland.

The pineal gland also produces melatonin, the hormone responsible for cell regeneration, having immunological properties that prevent cancer, heart disease, Alzheimer's and depression, among other illnesses, in addition to generating antioxidants that block free radicals responsible and regulate growth and puberty. Melatonin is scarce with insomnia and depression; therefore, a major cause of its loss lies in the manipulation of that which surrounds us; stress and anxiety are responsible for high levels of insomnia and depression, which minimize the activity of the pineal gland, generating a deficiency of not only DMT but of melatonin in our daily lives, leading to illnesses that submerge us further and further into the black hole of forgetting who we are.

Additionally, fluoride, now present in water, toothpaste, salt, and multiple foods, is one of the main factors responsible for calcifying, petrifying, and reducing the pineal gland, preventing spiritual growth of human beings and damaging our connection to other dimensions and the supreme essence of being, in other words, to the All. The importance of melatonin is obvious. We find this nutrient in foods such as oats, corn, tomatoes, potatoes, nuts, rice, cherries and, in extremely high doses, mangosteen. Beginning now, we will see how nutrition is a vital aspect of balance in our lives, health and spiritual growth.

Activating and developing the pineal gland allows us to break limiting ties and chains, filling historical emptiness and completely illuminating the path to be traveled, amplifying perspective of vision and human comprehension, to access our past and thus visualize and understand our future, connecting us to the entirety of our DNA, where the supreme essence is found, as well as all the wisdom of the universe. This turns us into integral beings, allowing us to vibrate outside of lineal time and space while we connect to our true self and the cosmos in a conscious manner, which banishes the darkness, occultism, and outer control. When we turn the light on, fears disappear and the chains of darkness are broken, leaving behind only freedom. True freedom is freedom from Point Zero, that singularity that allows us to create, welcoming Everything, impregnating everything with absolute unconditional love.

Accessing the light of ancestral knowledge is to be able to navigate the various dimensions, contacting the beings that live or belong in each of them, allows us to return to origin, to connect to Source, and it opens the path to elevate ourselves to high vibrational levels, connecting to the cosmos and the creator mind, accessing the true power that activates our supra-physical abilities and expand the perception of our mind and the vision of the third eye.

So we could say these dimensions are different levels of reality. As our vibrational frequencies elevate, our reality changes to a lighter density. The same thing happens to the consciousness; the higher the level of vibration, the easier it is to understand that we are consciousness. This goes beyond the concept of "reaching" it; we simply realize we are it.

The only formula that exists to heighten our levels of vibration and tune into much more elevated frequencies is to tune into the frequency of Love. Truly, love is the key to awakening. Rather than "awakening our consciousness," we "awake into consciousness." The concepts of vibration and frequency are explained in greater detail in chapter X.

Being conscious of this Inter-dimensionality makes us more sensitive and able to co-create a collective perception of any type of life, regardless of its form or location. It is in that place that a new form of cooperation begins.

Sometimes we believe that if we don't perceive something with our five senses, it doesn't exist. From that perspective, we can claim that UV rays don't exist because we cannot see them, or that ultrasounds do not exist because we do not hear them.

The dimensions are actually the various levels that our energy experiences in its evolutionary process toward Oneness. If we identify our inner energy as consciousness, we can say that dimensions are its different levels. The difference among them is the frequencies with which they vibrate.

In densities superior or lighter than 3D, we find what we call ascended masters, spiritual guides, angels and archangels. It is important to remember that these dimensions are in our DNA, not outside ourselves, and that we can access them through the evolution of consciousness. The moment we accept that we are multidimensional beings, we truly understand concepts such as the Superior Self, that part of ourselves found in higher planes of consciousness or dimensions. When we achieve a clear connection, we can make wise choices in every moment of our lives; furthermore, connecting to our Superior Self will free us from duality. We understand that it is not an expression separate from us, but another part of ourselves that allows us from the

Oneness, the Love and the Consciousness that we are, to see reality.

The Superior Self is our copilot on this journey called physical life, and it is what helps us evolve quickly. When we integrate ourselves entirely with its essence, we can access the unlimited Inter-dimensionality. One of the most powerful and important barriers to break down, in order to achieve that ideal communication and fusion, is the ego, which makes us believe that we are separate and alters our perception of time. This is why IRB considers the Higher Self the highest elevated essence of our being, and we emphasize that the Higher Self is our own essence existing on a higher level of consciousness, not another "I" separate from the "I" incarnate.

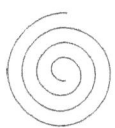

Chapter VII
Critical Mass

With this faith, we will be able to hew out of the mountain of despair a stone of hope. With this faith, we will be able to transform the jangling discords of our nation into a beautiful symphony of brotherhood. With this faith, we will be able to work together, to pray together, to struggle together, to go to jail together, to stand up for freedom together, knowing that we will be free one day.
Dr. Martin Luther King Jr.

The aforementioned Elite who are manipulating the world must always have some enemy from which to save us or protect us. In this way, they are able to keep our minds in the lower frequencies of fear, never seeing what is really happening. In other words, the key is to keep us distracted, fearing something or someone so that we do not wake up. It is much easier to govern people who are afraid, who believe the manipulation. For some, capitalists are the enemy; for others it's the communists, warlords, drug lords or terrorists. Sin, sickness and poverty are common factors in almost every society, to the point where we become immune to them, thinking they are normal.

When unconscious fear takes over, we fail to understand that the only way not to give power to the game of manipulation and war, the game of opposites, is not by losing or winning or taking sides

— the only way is by not playing the game. Every opposing side comes from the same source, part of the Whole.

While art and the media are great tools for creating consciousness, they are also used to give more power to the manipulators. For example, in 2012 we were made to believe that the world would end, that we had to protect ourselves from an extraterrestrial invasion. "They" were coming to conquer us, much like what happened in America with Christopher Columbus. The only true thing about that is that the metaphorical structures built by old beliefs are now crumbling down and giving way to a new reality. Before, the strategy was to create a problem until people reacted then generate a solution; just like those who create a virus and then the antivirus in a computer. Those who create one, create the other, in order to divide and conquer. But in the end, those who fight never win, though they want you to believe otherwise.

This is a transcendent moment in the history of the planet, as now there are many awakened people assisting in the transformation. The change does not happen on some specific date; it is already happening. We are living during the most important period of our civilization, planting the seeds of the New Earth. They key, as we have already seen, is to not go into the lower frequencies of fear, but rather to keep ourselves united in the frequency of love.

> IF ENOUGH PEOPLE UNDERSTAND THAT LOVE IS THE ONLY IMPORTANT THING IN LIFE, THEN WE CAN BECOME THE CRITICAL MASS THAT WILL GESTATE A NEW HUMANITY. LOVE IS THE WAY!

When we come to understand the infinite power of being connected to that part of the vital force, that frequency in which our creative faculties — aided by our thoughts, words, emotions and actions — help us become aware of the thought patterns that create a reality we have only dreamed of, a life without limits; in that moment, we radiate an expansive wave that inspires others. When focused on manifesting from Love rather than from fear, we are able to bring forth what we want from this vital force instead of what we don't want. There is no point in visualizing the life we would like to live, and endeavor to give power to our vision with thoughts and positive affirmation, if we continue to act upon our old patterns. This generates frustration, and we lose trust in our ability to change the world. It is at this point that we feel that our efforts are futile and so abandon them. We let the daily habits of our lives, of what we hear, settle into the collective consciousness that is stronger than what we imagine, scaring away the ideas we once dreamed of.

We are constantly being pulled by our fears and limiting beliefs that seem real, instead of giving power to our goals, dreams and creations. As a result, we feel frustration, things get worse, and our situation becomes more exasperating. We end up feeling completely disconnected and have a difficult time finding an exit. We must understand that reality is that which we manifest through focus and true intention. Everything is energy, vibration, and consciousness. When going deeper into quantum physics, we learn that when something reaches critical mass, a change occurs that cannot be stopped. It has been shown that if an electron increases its vibration until it has reached critical mass, it is unfailingly attracted to the highest frequency. It has been said that critical mass is fifty-one percent of the total of something. Going back to the electron, when its 51% vibrates at an elevated frequency, the 49% that remains is absorbed into the new frequency.

Since everything is energy and is made up of atoms, that theory also applies to our lives. Whenever we give power to what we think, say, feel, and sense may happen, at the moment that the 51% of our energy, vibration, and consciousness is synced with that belief, this reaches critical mass, and then nothing can stop this process.

Everything we manifest in our visible reality was first created in invisible reality, where it is merely information. Since our senses lead us to believe that only what we perceive through them is real, many times we give up before that 51% can occur. We back out one step before reaching critical mass. This is why sometimes our projects and visualizations do not manifest in the visible world.

Critical mass means that when we focus on creating wellbeing in our lives, the moment that our thoughts, words, emotions, and actions meet 51%, the circumstances in our lives change and we begin to experience perfection. If we continue to vibrate in the consciousness of fear, the negative critical mass takes us the opposite way. The moment that 51% of our focus tunes in to the frequency of Love, we become magnets for loving relationships. The moment that 51% of our focus tunes into peace, harmony, and balance, we manifest these tangible divine qualities in our life experiences.

Our divine potential is infinitely more powerful than illness, failure, dysfunctional relationships, hate, greed, corruption, war, or any other disturbance created by the manipulators that appear on the screen of everyday life.

When we devote our energy to facilitate the experiences that we want to create in our lives, and not the undesired experiences, we manifest our visions and dreams more quickly than we can possibly imagine. If this is possible for each of us, it is also possible that collectively, as a global family, we activate the New Jerusalem on Earth. To achieve this, it is fundamental to put things in perspective and accept the responsibility that we have as interconnected individuals to make this divine plan a reality.

If every day, every second, each of us puts forth only thoughts, words, actions and emotions that come from Love, which is the perfection we want to manifest in our lives, we will experience this change immediately. The transformation will become reality. Love is the sacred place where Zero Point exists, the matrix of Creation.

Up until now, a small group of people have been able to orchestrate the world's direction on a global scale, which we have had a hard time believing. Since it is impossible to control so many people physically, manipulation has been accomplished by distorting the way we think and feel until the desired behavior in people is achieved through mental and emotional manipulation. David Icke says:

> Herd Mentality: "We laugh at sheep because sheep just follow the one in front. We humans have out-sheeped the sheep, because at least the sheep need a sheep dog to keep them in line. Humans keep each other in line. And they do it by ridiculing or condemning anyone who commits the crime, and that's what it's become, of being different." (2009).

The expression "critical mass," besides coming from the aforementioned electron theory, comes from The Hundredth Monkey, by Ken Keyes, Jr., whose original excerpt was found in the book Lifetide by biologist Lyan Watson, published in 1979:

> The Japanese monkey Macaca Fuscata had been observed in the wild for a period of over thirty years. In 1952, on the island of Koshima, scientists were providing monkeys with sweet potatoes dropped in the sand. The monkey liked the taste of the raw sweet potatoes, but they found the dirt unpleasant. An eighteen-month-old female named Imo found she could solve the problem by washing the potatoes in a nearby stream. She taught this trick to her mother. Her playmates also learned this new way and they taught their mothers, too. This cultural innovation was gradually picked up by various monkeys before the eyes of the scientists. Between 1952 and 1958, all the young monkeys learned to wash the sandy sweet potatoes to make them more palatable. Only the adults who imitated their children learned this social improvement. Other adults kept eating the dirty sweet potatoes. Then something startling took place. In the autumn of 1958, a certain number of Koshima monkeys were washing sweet potatoes--the exact number is not known. Let us suppose that when the sun rose one morning there were ninety-nine monkeys on Koshima Island who had learned to wash their sweet potatoes. Let's further suppose that later that morning, the hundredth

monkey learned to wash potatoes. THEN IT HAPPENED! By that evening almost everyone in the tribe was washing sweet potatoes before eating them. The added energy of this hundredth monkey somehow created an ideological breakthrough! But notice: A most surprising thing observed by these scientists was that the habit of washing sweet potatoes then jumped over the sea...Colonies of monkeys on other islands, and on the mainland troop of monkeys at Takasakiyama, began washing their sweet potatoes.

This means that even though we do not know the exact number of people it takes to achieve critical mass, the phenomenon of the hundredth monkey scientifically proves that when a certain number of people know a new method, it becomes conscious property of the group. And when one more person tunes into the new knowledge, it will reach the entire world, just as, in the excerpt above, more and more monkeys began to learn the new behavior until, one fine day, the entire colony was washing their sweet potatoes. What is perhaps most surprising is that, starting from that day, other monkeys in other islands, without contact from those before, also learned to wash their sweet potatoes, as if the new knowledge had gone through the air, affecting the entire species. Watson concluded that when a certain number of monkeys learned this behavior, critical mass was reached. In other words, we had the required number of monkeys for the entire species to learn this new knowledge or behavior. And something even more important to note is that the one who brought the change was a young female monkey. We adults have a tendency to repeat old patterns, which means it is very important to listen to the youth, to the new generations, instead of criticizing, reprimanding, or pigeonholing them into what has always been done. They bring the information for change, and it is important, more than teaching them, to learn from them.

This means that in the evolution of the species there are mechanisms that affect the way that ideas and customs spread throughout the whole species. This was called "the theory of the hundredth monkey." Watson confirmed in his book that if a large enough number of people — the critical mass, fifty-one percent — acquires a new understanding or way of seeing things, this propagates to all of humanity; that means that it only takes one person to complete the critical mass and trigger a new understanding for humans.

> ARE YOU THE HUNDREDTH MONKEY? OR
> ARE YOU GOING TO CONTINUE TO FOLLOW
> WHAT THE OTHERS WANT YOU TO DO?
> SYNC TO IRB
> SO THAT PLANET EARTH MAY FIND BALANCE

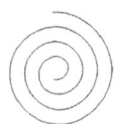

Chapter VIII
Teachers or Gods?

The gap that has been produced by the great work to our surroundings is a good place to light our little light. This is where geniuses come from, the universal inspiration that pushes us beyond imitation.

Franz Kafka

Throughout human history we have seen many teachers and many gods. One of the main individuals to hold both titles, Jesus of Nazareth, marked our civilization to such an extent that history divides itself into before (B.C.) and after (A.D. or C.E.) Christ. The latter stands for anno domini: "in the year of the Lord." Jesus was such an exceptional being, as we mentioned in Chapter IV, that delving into his life seems almost redundant. However, in this section it is essential to the understanding of our existence on Earth and the power we have over it, to bring up this admirable being's history.

As part of the manipulation that has us believing that God is an entity separate from us whom we must worship, Catholicism imprints God's nature, and the role of God's only son, upon Jesus the Christ, which completely misrepresents his time on Earth. Now millions of people worship Jesus as a God instead of accepting his teaching that we are all God.

Jesus as a teacher invites us to learn from him and encourages us to believe that, if we can be like him, or even better, when he says, "Whoever believes in me will also do the works that I do; and greater works than these will he do." (John 14:12)

What magic works did Jesus do in his public life? He walked on water, healed the sick, gave sight to the blind, resuscitated the dead, multiplied bread and fish, and turned water into wine. How is it then possible that we, simple mortals that we are, can do greater things than those? Where is the secret that gives us superhuman powers?

Jesus came to summarize the ten commandments of Moses into one: "Love one another As I have loved you." (John 13:34) The secret is very simple; it has been there for years: when we are pure Love, we do not need laws to follow because we become the law. There is nothing that Love cannot achieve, there is nothing that Love can damage. The frequency of Love is the highest vibrational frequency in the universe. All we have to do is tune into this powerful frequency to obtain the divine power and knowledge to fully connect to Source.

Besides bringing in this frequency, Jesus gave us a prayer that we can repeat unceasingly, which itself can create a miracle. In the Lord's Prayer, Jesus declares that we are all children of God, which makes us one with the Father, One with All that Is, in equality and brotherhood. This prayer encapsulates Jesus' teaching that the ultimate aim is Love, not religion.

Jesus wrote the Lord's Prayer when he was fourteen years old, by which time Joseph had died and Jesus had become the head of the household. It is said that Jesus had discussions with his mother, Mary, about the Jewish teaching that we must oppose evil. This was a cornerstone belief that Jesus questioned, prompting him to teach that our actions must come from Love and the joy of being one with the universal Father. The Lord's Prayer has become iconic, and philosophies such as metaphysics, pranic healing, and others, have taken apart this prayer and made it a scientific postulate. Below we go over each phrase and summarize some of the truths each reveals. IRB divides this scientific formula into three paragraphs:

1. Our Father: In this opening, we establish our true divine nature and where we came from. We understand that we are spiritual beings. We are what is represented by figures such as Christ, Buddha, and Krishna. We are children of God, made in his image and greatness; we have in our genes the divine gene. Note that Jesus says "our Father," not "my Father," which shows that we are all children of the same father and that he is not the only son of God.

2. Who art in Heaven: "Heaven" refers to the inner world, and, as was explained thoroughly in Chapter IV, our thoughts can create an inner state of Love that is Heaven itself. If the Father is within us, then we must not look for him outside ourselves in a temple, church, or synagogue. It is in our inner reflections that He resides permanently. This invites us to recognize the Presence of God in all that exists, including what we consider empty space. Even there, life manifests in dimensions undetected by our physical senses. Besides, we understand that if everything is God, Heaven is not only inside ourselves and our thoughts, which means we can personally experience Heaven, but we can also turn any external event into Heaven, depending on how we choose to look at it.

3. Hallowed be thy name: Whatever comes out of our minds and mouths must be good and healthy. That is the meaning behind the saying, "What comes out of your mouth is more important than what goes into it." If what we put into our mouths is contaminated, it contaminates our soul and generates contaminated thoughts. Since thought is the original spark of any creation, whatever we create from it can either be clean and pure, or contaminated. This phrase invites us to be responsible for the creative power of words: therefore, it is important to be careful with what we think and say, since everything materializes. When we say, "I am," and follow it with an insult, we are no longer hallowing the name, which is our Presence.

4. Thy kingdom come: This phrase emphasizes the Love energy that comes through virtues such as compassion, mercy, giving and sharing. Through giving and sharing, we generate prosperity and abundance, inheriting the kingdom. This is the main secret to prosperity and richness. We create the consciousness that we are always stepping onto sacred ground because we belong in Eden, in Paradise, where there is never illness or lack. Everything is God, so we live in his kingdom. It is Love that rules the kingdom and dictates the code of conduct.

5. Thy will be done: Walking the spiritual path means synchronizing the power of our inferior human nature with the will of our superior expression, or our divine nature. This phrase means to activate and augment our inner strength under the influence of the supreme essence of our Christ nature with direct connection to Source.

6. On Earth as it is in Heaven: Good thoughts, good words, good feelings, and good will, must all manifest in good actions. This phrase reveals the secret of greater physical energy, which is necessary for the evolution of the physical body as a vessel for a highly evolved being; it offers us the knowledge of the magnitude of the universe, understanding that everything is guided by the one universal law of infinity. As human beings, we are The Zero Point, the point from which inner and outer expand and Heaven on Earth is created.

7. Give us this day our daily bread: This phrase has been highly manipulated, and for many years we were made to believe that we had to ask in order to receive, that we had to beg and feel as if we cannot receive by our own means, but there is someone of higher status who must give it to us. This phrase is one of the most powerful in the prayer. The word "bread" is a symbol of the vital energy that the physical body requires in order to live, which is also known as mana, *chi, ki,* or *prana.* We know that bread remains fresh for one day only, so we are invited us to live in the present, which is the whole key to consciousness. The eternal present invites us to break through the linear concept of time and, with each decision, to live in loving acceptance of the creative instant, which is unique and unrepeatable. This is also a loving act, for it speaks in plural form: not of mine and yours, but of ours, of something belonging to us all, which is proof that everything is given to us even before we ask for it, and when we manifest for everyone, we receive proportionally, as we too are part of the Whole.

8. Forgive us our trespasses, as we forgive those who trespass against us: This is the original phrase twisted by fear, being changed over time to mean "forgive offenses." It is important to understand that there can be no offense against us. Every situation we experience we create ourselves so that we can learn and grow, and every "offense" is actually a gift from a teacher we chose along our path of evolution. Besides, no one can hurt us if we don't allow them to. No one can "give" offense; that is merely an interpretation from our own perspective of events. Furthermore, it is important to accept that the only thing that is offended is our ego; nothing cannot offend our Presence. From a state of deep Presence, the only possible experience is the acceptance of perfection, of the divine plan. Our true essence, our inner energy, can never be offended or harmed, since it is perfect. So this phrase is truly powerful, being pure alchemy, capable of transforming lead into gold; it generates inner healing, transforming what seems a destructive, violent, volatile situation into understanding, harmony and peace from a place of Love. Love is the real instrument of forgiveness, which in reality is simply accepting our own responsibility for every situation.

9. And lead us not into temptation, but deliver us from evil: On the one hand, this phrase refers to the sexual power we discussed in Chapter IV. Sex is natural and healthy. Creational or generative sexual energy can be transmuted into superior creative power. The desire for physical union can become divine union with Source. This phrase refers to transmutation of sexual energy into regenerative energy, loving energy, creative energy, and divine energy. The transmutation of sexual energy is vital for spiritual development. Transmuted sexual energy provides energy that nourishes body and mind, meaning our whole being. Unfortunately, more than anything else, sexual energy has manipulated the human race, completely confining and limiting our powers of manifestation. Temptation lies in fomenting sexuality for genital pleasure alone. In reality, sexual energy is the quintessential creative force through which we manifest projects, wellbeing, health, or any other situation we wish to create through Love — the energy that that makes us divine unlimited beings. On the other hand, temptation also means not allowing superficiality and appearances of the things of the world to deceive us. Only by doing this can we free ourselves from all that hinders our growth. The greatest temptation we have in daily life is to fail to remember our divine power.

10. For yours is the kingdom: This phrase and the one that follows were eliminated from the prayer since, coming at the end of the prayer, they give enormous power to human expression when said in full awareness. This refers to the understanding and ascension of Kundalini, or the serpent of the sacred fire in our being. Spiritual energy descends from this Kundalini energy in order to awaken and ascend to the sacred field of universal wisdom, manifesting both as an expansion of consciousness.

11. The power and the glory: This phrase allows us to activate the inner vessel that connects us to the multi-dimensional. It reveals our power to access any type of information, in any place, in any universe, and from whichever teacher, at any level of consciousness we have created. By accessing this power to create from the union of divine inner will and external human will, we access glory, where there is only ecstasy and abundance.

12. Forever and ever: This phrase connects us with infinity, with timelessness, and with the maximum power of creation. When we recognize ourselves as unlimited beings, we access the multi-dimensional and live in an illuminated way.

13. Amen: This is the most powerful seal of manifestation; it means it is done, and so be it.

When we continue to analyze Jesus as one of the greatest teachers ever witnessed by humanity, it is quite strange that none of the stories in the sacred scriptures cover his life from the ages of twelve to thirty. According to the Bible, Jesus spent those thirty years making tables and chairs with his father Joseph. Documents exist that reveal the actual spiritual preparations that Jesus underwent during those years, to ready him for his last three years on Earth. The *Urantia Book* is one of such documents. In 1887, the Russian journalist Nicolas Notovitch discovered some manuscripts in Buddhist monasteries in Ladakh that confirm that, between the ages of twelve and thirty, Jesus traveled to India, Ladakh, Tibet and even Egypt, where he trained to impart his greatest teachings. The omission of this information is just part of the manipulation. The Bible as we know it was edited by order of Roman Emperor Constantine. Some historians confirm that the emperor specifically ordered all Evangelical texts referring to Jesus' more human side to be omitted, emphasizing instead those that focused on his Divinity.

How can it be that Constantine, who was never a Christian and was baptized on his death bed, should be the one to omit essential aspects of Christ's teachings? An example among many others is the omission of the concept of reincarnation, which most Christians believed at the time. This means that the Gospels that attest to the story of Jesus were manipulated by the political interests of the time. To get a better understanding of the subject, watch the documentary How Jesus Became a Christ: The Hidden Years, based on Miceal Ledwith's lifelong study of available sources.

However, if we look beyond the question of whether Jesus' life is truthfully told, or whether he learned in other countries, what remains clear is that Jesus's central teaching, one that contains all the information we need to change our reality: The Love commandment. Love is not just a feeling we express to people who are nice to us, nor does it mean that we must love our enemies. Love goes beyond that ephemeral understanding. When we connect with the energy of Love, we imitate Master Jesus in all his dimensions, in the entirety of his creative powers. We understand the miracles of daily life. When we act fully conscious of our divine Presence, we awaken to our true estate. To Love one another is the teaching of the master and the key that opens the door to the new world that began, according to Mayan prophecy, on December 21, 2012. At that moment, our planet perfectly aligned with our Sun and with the center of our galaxy, referred to as *Hunab Ku* by the Mayans. This alignment creates a very powerful energy with a high vibration that generates the feeling of Love. That is the key to living in the new galactic dawn that we will be consolidating for in the next 26,000 years on the new Earth.

There are many who have demonstrated through science that Love has a high and rapid frequency, and that fear has a very low, sloth-like frequency. Above all, it is important to understand that fear is the antithesis of Love. If we wish to benefit from the high energy generated by this new galactic dawn, it is important to vibrate at the frequency of Love, understanding that We Are All One, that we are the manifestation of Source on Earth. Acting from our mastery enables us to live, love and create as Gods. Why would we want to love? To activate 100% of our DNA, just as the great masters and avatars have done. To create from our divinity a universe that is harmonious and balanced, with equality for all, as so many have wished for throughout history. This can only be achieved through the consciousness that emerges from a fully potentiated DNA.

Chapter IX
Where Are We Headed?

You can create 'today' the events of your 'tomorrow'
Helena Blavatsky

How interesting it is to see a compass needle point toward one direction, no matter how it's positioned: Earth's magnetic North! It is known that there are two north poles: the magnetic north indicated by this interesting little gadget that, no matter what, never loses orientation; and the geographic north, the actual axis around which the Earth rotates. These two poles do not coincide and are increasingly distancing themselves from each other, to the point where the magnetic north pole will end up being, at some point in the future, at the geographic south pole of the Earth. This means that time as we know it in 3D is radically changing, becoming shorter in duration. As I write this book, our twenty-four-hour day is actually fourteen hours long, which is why we have the feeling that time is moving much faster. This reversal of the magnetic poles is said to have begun in December of 2012.

The way to understand this is more or less the same as understanding how the energetic vortexes of the human body spin. There are moments when they turn clockwise and others when they turn counter-clockwise. The Earth, too, is a vortex and behaves as such. So its rotation is slowing down and will eventually move in the opposite direction. As the Earth's electromagnetic field decreases, its vibrational frequency increases. This frequency is known as the Schumann Resonance, which has been dubbed the heartbeat of the planet. According to the scale created by the German physicist Winfried Otto Schumann, the highest number assigned to the magnetic field is one and the lowest thirteen, which would be the point where the earth stops its rotation. For many centuries, this value was 7.8Hz, but it began to increase in frequency in 1980. Today it is close to twelve cycles per second, which could mean that our planet is one step away from ceasing its rotation. I am still not sure whether that would occur physically or metaphorically, but it is important to remember this information to understand the importance of the number thirteen, which is reflected in the thirteenth layer of our DNA, as in Zero Point energy, a subject we will touch upon later.

On our planet, according to the Gregorian Calendar, one day lasts twenty-four hours divided by day and night. The Mayans confirmed that one galactic day lasts 25,625 earth years — rounded up to 26,000 — and it is also divided into day and night. This means that one galactic day or night would equal 12,812 years. The twenty-first of December, 2012, was the end of 12,812 years of darkness, or night. At that point we entered what has been called the Dawn of the Galaxy. That cosmic event coincides with the end of the Mayan Long Count calendar, and the alignment of the Earth with the Sun, and simultaneously the center of the Milky Way, as previously mentioned.

During that whole time of darkness — which I like to call "winter," as a galactic season of cold and darkness — our planet was far away from the center of the Milky Way; in other words, we were all but disconnected from that center that generates one of the highest vibrations. Because of this, various methods have been developed over time to try to re-connect with that potent energy. This is the reason we created the spiritual tools and techniques we know today.

There are many theories and prophecies, such as that of the Hopi, Padre Pio, Nostradamus, and Apocalypse among others, that confirm that the Earth will soon go through a period of three days of darkness. It is very likely that this period is due to the pause that the Earth undergoes when it reverses its rotation. Beyond what may happen in these three days of darkness, it is likely that Earth, Gaia, along with the human race and other beings that populate it, will undergo a great transformation. It is important to be aware that as the earth increases its vibrational frequencies, our cells —which also vibrate — will synchronize to the new rhythm of vibration on our planet, which will affect our emotions and, most of all, our DNA.

> FOR EARTH TO STOP ROTATING
> MEANS TO PRACTICALLY PRODUCE
> ZERO POINT

The chaos that allows for building anew

What awaits us in the next 26,000 thousand years? A new dawn filled with Love and Living Light.

If where we are now is the dawn of the galaxy, "the spring," why then do we still need the candles we used for lighting the nocturnal path where we then found ourselves? The spiritual tools that we have counted on until now have been small guiding lights. They were at our service to light the path that took us to the Source of energy that, in the long galactic night, was very far away. Now that we are in the era of Living Light, we no longer need these tools. What help can a small candle offer in the broad light of day? As the cycle of Love and Living Light that illuminates everything begins, we no longer need anything outside ourselves to light the way. Still we must be grateful for the tools that helped us during times of darkness and disconnection. We now begin the cycle of recognition of our own power through Love, which creates everything and is the life in each cell and atom. No longer shall we surrender our power to external factors. THIS IS THE TIME to trust that we are light, color, sound, number and geometry, the carriers of absolute knowledge; this is the time to recognize ourselves as our own teachers, completely connected to divine essence. To this end, we must simply make the decision to connect to this new frequency from Zero Point, which is available to everyone, to regain access to the Source.

> IRB IS A TOOL CREATED IN THE NEW ENERGY,
> AVAILABLE TO ALL
> WITHOUT COMPLICATIONS. IT IS A DIRECT CONNECTION
> TO THE LIVING LIGHT, LOVE, AND SOURCE.
> IT IS THE CONSCIOUSNESS THAT DISTANCES US FROM FEAR
> AND BRINGS US CLOSER TO LOVE
> FROM THE SACRED SILENCE OF SELF.

To accompany the Earth in this process is an individual decision and, as always, amenable to free will. If the decision is to evolve our consciousness to the multi-dimensional, it is very important that our inner compass be perfectly aligned to the pole of Love and not that of fear. Meditation and breathing are very powerful tools for achieving this.

> IRB, THE COMPLETE CHANGE OF CONSCIOUSNESS TO ACTIVATE
> IN EACH BEING THE ELECTROMAGNETIC FIELD
> THAT ALLOWS THE DEFINITE SYNCING TO LOVE, ZERO POINT, AND THE
> CHRIST CONSCIOUSNESS IN THE TOTALITY OF OUR DNA

Chapter X
The Original Model

In the classical theory of general relativity [...] the principle of the universe must be a singularity of density and curvature of space/time. In these circumstances, all known laws of physics cease to govern.

Stephen William Hawking

Cinematography is one of the main tools evolved beings can use to activate our Conscious selves and slowly introduce ourselves to a new reality. My favorite film, The Matrix (1999, written and directed by Larry and Andy Wachowski), is an almost seven-hour-long trilogy that explains the human situation very clearly; for many years we have been submerged in an illusion on one side of a veil of secrecy, but we can find our "Original Model" through a simple shift in consciousness. I vividly remember Morpheus offering Neo the two pills: the blue one that would allow him to remain a slave to the Matrix, or the red one that would allow him to awaken to his true self, his true potential. IRB is that red pill! It allows us to find our true potential and recognize our true origin. It permits us to leave behind the illusion that for years we have called reality; it lets us transcend the five senses, as mentioned in Chapter IV.

The five senses have limited us to the point of making us believe that only what we perceive through them, exists. This is almost like a blind person saying that light or colors do not exist simply because he or she cannot see them. This is where our beliefs come in: we are what we believe. Beliefs are our operating system.

Another film that touches on the subject of beliefs is the movie Life Is Beautiful (1997, written and directed by Roberto Benigni). In the plot, a father entirely changes the reality of World War II for his son by making him believe that their lives in a concentration camp is a game. The game of life changes based on how we perceive it.

There is ample information on the topic of belief, thanks to copious amounts of professions and techniques in healing and reprogramming that lead us to make fundamental changes to live better. Yet this, too, is but a dim candle that barely illuminates our journey in the 3D world, since it leads us to the understanding of different personal realities. The truth is that the only way to live in peace and harmony is by respecting each other's reality.

What if, from this change on, what we gain is the understanding of the truth that we must completely transcend into a new paradigm? It is not about changing to a paradigm where, one way or another, we once again create as before and generate a new collective consciousness, because this means anchoring ourselves again to limits, new limits that are perhaps less limiting, but limits nonetheless. The Truth is Freedom without limits, and this is the understanding of being Consciousness.

We have already talked about how science states that everything that exists is energy, and that energy is composed of atoms that vibrate at a certain frequency, based on the state they find themselves in. 99.9% of the atom is empty space, based on the atomic model of Rutherford, who in 1911, along with Geiger and Marsden, confirmed this reality in different experiments. To explain it without going too far into scientific terminology, we will say that various states of matter result from the frequency at which the atoms vibrate.

If the frequency is low, the matter is more solid. If the frequency is high, the matter is less dense, and it's our cells that determine that, based on stored memories. Our brain generates thoughts based on these memories, which on their own, produce associated emotions. Something very important to the changing of our reality is to be 100% conscious of the responsibility we have over our thoughts, our words, our feelings, and our actions, so they can be consistent and thus create a stable reality.

Before a manifestation occurs on the physical plane, it begins as energy so subtle we cannot see it, but it creates a particular vibration based on the frequency at which it is emitted. The thoughts that we call positive generally vibrate at a higher frequency, just as negative thoughts vibrate at lower frequencies. According to the vibration or frequencies we tune into, so is the reality we create. When the majority of people are tuned to the same frequency, we achieve the critical mass discussed in a previous chapter; the collective beliefs become a reality for the majority, whether in our region or on the entire planet. The higher we vibrate, the more access we have to superior realities.

Transforming our limiting beliefs of separation, superiority, or inferiority into the absolute certainty that We Are All One, leads us to the development of respect for all manifestations of life. Just by changing our beliefs, it is possible to generate a new paradigm of unity as a collective and access the Truth.

When we manage to understand that Love is the only possible power, and that if we vibrate in tune with it we are invulnerable, we connect to Source and rediscover our true essence which is stored in the thirteenth layer of our DNA, which we will talk about in depth later.

Living with the understanding of this responsibility allows us to change the direction of our evolution. Cosmic events cause changes in the terrestrial magnetic fields and, in consequence, change the neural fields of the human brain and our cells, causing major shifts in consciousness.

Dieter Duhm (2012) confirmed that, thanks to the new models of perception and thought, new concepts of conviviality are arising, including a new relationship between the sexes based on truth and trust. Now sexuality is no longer connected to the collective trauma of fear and violence, but rather gratitude and joy. New paths are being carved for Love which, after a longstanding history of war, are being unblocked. Far and wide across the world, the strength of transparency and of the Christ impulse are manifesting, allowing us to find a structure for inner healing which is stored in our DNA. This is where we will make contact with the Original Mode, which permits the changing of the reality of our civilization. This process is the intended goal of every civilization.

When we all come together from our Original Model, we expand to the point of connection to the matrix of the planet, and form a single unified matrix, achieving that great peace which we have dreamed of for eons, which will finally become a reality, allowing us to reconnect with Source. That will result in the recovery of our genetic healing powers that come from the holon, to which the Earth, humans, and all livings beings are connected.

Breathing and meditation are quite important for the activation of our Original Model, since it is necessary to slow the neural frequency patterns to change the way we receive and respond to the information from the outside world. We must listen to our own inner alpha frequency sounds to extend the time segments and strengthen the rhythm of our exhalation. This is the way to rid the body of shields and unblock the lower abdomen and the life centers that reside there. The human DNA layers that have previously been locked will be activated.

When we come to a deep understanding of the thirteenth layer of our DNA, we begin to experience a profound change in the relationship between life and death, the here and the beyond; we manifest the eternal frequency that vibrates in the depth of this new state of consciousness and more easily perceive the information coming from the transcendental spaces of the world since the organs of perception are freed from the five senses and open to the unlimited influences of the universe.

The new dimension of consciousness activated by the Original Model is not limited to the spiritual field. It allows us to see ourselves as a whole, including fundamental aspects of the physical body, of sensory existence, and of energetic incorporation to the totality of life. With the activation of subtle energies, the material world changes, becoming lighter. The changes are more obvious in the area of sexuality and related dogmas, in the strengthening of feminine energy, the removing of the shield that separates us from the All, in the development of true trust between the sexes, in a new relationship with animals, and in a new connection with the great family of life. The duality between the body and the spirit that hinders the contact and comprehension among beings dissolves. Activating our Original Model allows for a natural vibration of coexistence to emerge, along with empathy and solidarity with all of creation in a frequency of unity that marks the new consciousness and the new basis of the New Earth. The holon, unity, is no longer just a philosophical term but rather an experience that allows us to take the existential leap.

The activation of our Original Model also makes it possible to change our inner structures to such a point that by changing our old thought structures we can modify history and humanity's collective pain from centuries of war, destruction, and hate.

The collective models of fear and violence are at the base of the current civilization. When fear dominates us, pain generates violence, creating a vicious cycle in which we become more manipulated and genetically create a neural legacy based on dogmatic structures that create patterns of behavior based on beliefs: "We must avenge what has happened;" "we must fight the battle;" "where there is jealousy there is love;" and many other phrases. These make up "hell," judgment and revenge, in which we have been submerged in this dense 3D world, and which are the bases for humanity's daily suffering.

The activation of the Original Model creates new neuro-pathways in the brain and changes the information inside the cell's nucleus and our DNA; thus, we can begin with new perceptions, new images and new impulses in our power commands, which we will discuss later. Patterns for self-healing, happiness, Unity and Love are activated as something inherent and natural, which leads to the practice of self-mastery.

This transformation is not always automatically and immediately evident. At the beginning there can be a clash between new and old beliefs, creating turbulence. The manipulative elite is trying to prevent the renovation of humanity, and those who feel comfortable in the old energy might rebel against new behaviors. Only Love can minimize the trauma by allowing the critical mass to achieve renovation in a simpler way, since the transformation comes from the connection and union with the superior Original Model supported by the universe.

A change in consciousness and respect toward all forms of life does not imply that we must embrace a vegetarian diet to avoid feeding our body with the low vibrations of death. Rather, we must begin by acknowledging and respecting beings such as ants, flies, rats, and so many others, that we have labeled as pests. We have invented poisons to eliminate them, ignoring that each of them, as manifestations of life on earth and in the universe, carries valuable information in our biological system, no matter how insignificant they may seem. Not unlike humans, they are also organs within the grand creature of life.

As mentioned briefly in Chapter VI, the importance of water is fundamental to the coming change, especially in the activation of our original model. Water is life in liquid form, and our physical bodies are composed of seventy-five percent water. Therefore, water is an excellent healing force and contains all the information of life that can help us attune to higher frequencies. When we drink water that is not genetically modified the way big industries have been doing, we can access one of the main carriers of information. The different forms of water on our planet, both on its surface and beneath it, are conduits of communication that bring us new information, which is why it is vital to consume her in her purest state. The new ecology that springs from our Original Model is a planetary ecology that allows us to work from a planetary and cosmic unity, to the point of making water emerge on its own. The times of water shortage, drought and desertification will end forever when we cooperate from the frequency of Love with nature.

Between the body of the Earth and the human body is a deep connection. Sexual energy is the purest conduit of this connection. As a result of a congestion of the flow of vital energies, our bodies tremble as when an infection takes hold of the human body and causes febrile shivering, or chills, as its visible manifestation. Likewise, the Earth manifests these shivers as earthquakes, volcanic eruptions and floods. In humanity, it manifests as diseases, psychoses, and violent outbursts. If we avoid human catastrophes, we avoid terrestrial and universal catastrophes.

By freeing man of the ghost of the conflicts of the past, we develop a new civilization in which energies align; both earthly and cosmic, both sexual and spiritual, all in harmony.

Proof that our original model is activated is when we access the feminine; it begins with the release of collective patterns that impede our ability to think and act from the feminine model. By reconnecting with Source, we recognize the absolute power of the feminine and see it expanding to the whole world; women rediscover their true role in creation and man activates his deepest sense of intuition.

With its gentle power, the feminine disintegrates hard structures, and new energetic fields are generated for Love and solidarity among beings. Men allow themselves to be accepted by women without having to adopt chauvinistic disguises; their purpose ceases to be that of fighting, conquest, and war. When the war between the sexes ends, all war will end.

Our physical body and our surroundings become subtler and more transparent; we understand the magic of the world being moved by, not only physical energy but mental and spiritual energies, as well. This is why from the Divine Consciousness of our Original Model, we can create a world through the mind that is unified by our heart, in a quick and easy way, starting from the strongest expressions that offer us the most results in limitless research into art, science, and spirituality.

Love then turns into a universal power with frequencies that heal old wounds — or better yet, syncs us into the information of the Field, where wounds are no longer useful, so that collective denial wrought by a long history of war becomes a collective affirmation. The collective memory will be one, and humanity will synchronize with the superior level of its only Source, with the most profound connection to all living beings, toward Oneness, toward the Divinity manifested in all of Creation.

With our Original Model, the cosmic connects to the terrestrial, the mental to the physical, the Marian with the sexual, the Christ-like with the political, the scientific with the mythological, the technological with the artistic, and thus all opposites unify from Zero Point in the great neutrality of Love. From these connections, new compositions are made: Eastern mysticism combines with Western science, Hopis with Europeans, shamans with modern specialists of high-end technology, and all types of musicians creating a universal symphony from Jerusalem to Tibet.

By connecting the thirteenth layer of our DNA, whose primary function is to orchestrate in a quantum fashion all the other layers that have been reconnected through healing processes, we create a new world without fear or war through the totality of our Original Model.

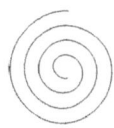

Chapter XI
We Are One

— Namaste —

*Every relationship is one of give and take.
To give inspires receiving, and to receive inspires giving.*

Deepak Chopra

In the traditional Mayan salute is a wonderful mantra referencing unity. One Mayan greets the other with *In Lak'ech,* (I am your other you), to which the other replies, Ala K'in, (You are me). Here is a complete recognition of unity and brotherhood. How can we hurt someone who is part of who we are?

We have referenced the existence of various dimensions. When we want to understand the dimensions superior to 3D, we can explain it in two ways: the first is by applying quantum physics, the second by using exclusively spiritual concepts. Although quantum physics and spirituality seem to describe contradictory worlds, they are just two languages that arrive at the same truth. Quantum physicists are using scientific language to explain the spiritual world, which for many years was viewed strictly as a religious topic.

Quantum physics study the behavior of mass and energy at an atomic and subatomic level. Works like *The Field* by Lynne McTaggart, *The Reconnection* by Eric Pearl, and the movie What the bleep Do We Know?! by William Arntz, are just a few examples of artists using quantum terms to approach spirituality.

We talked about ego in Chapter VI. How do we identify ego? The ego is the part of us that generates ideas of individuality; it makes us feel superior or inferior to others; it leads us to identify with matter; it feeds our body with pain through our emotions; it activates old memories stored in our cellular memory; it blocks the connection to the most elevated essence of our being; and it makes us forget that in truth we are Presence. One of the most effective ways to silence the inner voices that often confuse us and drive the separatist ego is meditation, or inner silence, which is the purest inner sound. When we can listen to our silence, we are able to achieve the connection with Source. When we connect to Source, we connect to Presence, to all that is; and by All Being One, every particle becomes a cosmos.

Nevertheless, to activate our Unity Consciousness, we must recognize and accept fear as the dark side of the *yin-yang* duality and realize that it is part of the whole and the perfect totality. Fear and its variations (hate, revenge, envy, resentment, pain, anxiety, sadness, and depression, among others) have been great teachers. Now this is the time to simply observe them from Love so as to no longer generate more of the same or allow them to continue to be the instruments of manipulation that keep us from observing truly. We do not have to resort to facing the events and what these vibrational fears have stored in our subconscious. We must only unify opposites, accepting the paradox and dichotomy, live in unity and neutrality, incorporate learning, and connect to new information from a place of Love, which is All. Love does not reject; Love welcomes, teaches, and learns in an eternal and infinite flow; allowing us to be permanent teachers and students of consciousness. Permanence is the present moment, and the present moment is Presence.

IRB is that consciousness of alchemical transformation that allows us to definitively transform fear into Love without forgetting who we are, but rather remember our divine essence, opening us to the infinite possibilities that connect us to the Zero Point Field. There, everything that exists is sustained by Love as possible and achievable without interference, for each of us. We simply activate the alchemic transmutation of consciousness toward life and true purpose.

Evolution is not individual; it is not even racial or societal; evolution is planetary. As we evolve as human beings, each natural and vital element that makes up the planet also evolves. Earth as a planet has a collective consciousness to which we connect through this evolution process, which, in this chapter, we will now call metamorphosis.

The work, however, is individual. This transformation from caterpillar to butterfly is an individual one, consciously transforming low-frequency, fear-based emotions into solidarity, friendship, and service to others, activating total Compassion.

Achieving this timelessness, living this "time without time," being here without experiencing hurry, understanding that time is also One with Everything, we can accept that living and dying are only temporary existential phases, for we were, and are, and will continue to be. That is true freedom. The timelessness of the wise man who contemplates human complications without being affected, since his spirit is in that paradise that offers wonderful inner peace that continues now and forever in Presence. We must heed the teachings of the great masters of our spiritual history such as Eckhart Tolle and Osho, and lower the number of trips through time (from past to future and vice versa) where we waste precious energy that is needed for our metamorphosis.

It is imperative that we heal our addiction to a future that persuades us to postpone joy and freedom until tomorrow. Why wait when we can enjoy them today? Nothing can replace the simple joy of being fully present in even the most mundane acts of daily life, such as feeding ourselves, brushing our teeth, walking on the street, or any other daily activity.

Likewise, it is important to recognize the outmoded reality that still surrounds us, a result of our historical disconnection from consciousness, so as to not allow exterior factors to affect our mood and inner peace. The outer world can be like a hurricane, its intensity and magnitude becoming greater and greater. Placing ourselves in the eye of the hurricane allows us to enjoy silence, calm, and serenity, even in the middle of the maelstrom, because there singularity lies, at the Zero Point, which allows us to create in full consciousness.

From that state of peace, we can direct our energy, not toward fighting what is already outdated and obsolete in the heart, but toward creating from the newness that lives in every heartbeat. It is therefore essential to end the addiction to the media and fear-based discussions regarding the conflicts, crises and countless controversies happening in the outside world. We must take on the challenge to be free, to remove ourselves from the virtual prison we've put ourselves in. We have created prison bars out of fear, false responsibilities, guilt, limiting beliefs, judgments, control, and all that the ego demands in order to fulfill its need for acknowledgment, security, and protection.

THIS IS THE TIME for freedom. Freedom is not what humanity has idealized in its mind; freedom is the absolute absence of fear. Fear is replaced in the heart by complete trust in life and its events, in its perfection, and in the innate knowledge of our shared and quantum DNA, where we accept from our consciousness that nothing has to change because everything is perfect!

Many people ask me, "What happens to 3D when the metamorphosis is complete? Does it disappear?" The 3D world, just like everything up to this point has its reason for being and will always exist as part of creation, just like an unused musical note will always exist as part of the musical scale. We cannot pretend to eliminate it or even change it. It is a matter of fully accepting that nothing has to change because everything is perfect! Everything goes together and has its place in the cosmos and creation, including the 3D world where we have spent thousands of years developing our vital experiences and the experiences of our consciousness. Life and consciousness are One, the fruit of Love, their genesis.

The only difference between old energy and new energy is that something drives us to live and vibrate differently. The metamorphosis does not come from the need to change the 3D world, but from an inner need to evolve and create from infinite Love, with which we can access the totality of the present, wherever we choose to experience it. 3D is part of the information and the path that we currently choose to follow; it brings us valuable information and, just like the rest, exists in our DNA. Within perfection, nothing needs to be rejected, nothing is invalid, and nothing is destroyed.

This is why IRB, more than a change, is an alchemical and evolutionary metamorphosis that comes from within and radiates to the outside, to share with all humans, Mother Earth, and all other creatures. A caterpillar undergoing metamorphosis into a butterfly does not propose changes to its surroundings. It doesn't dwell on what it cannot accept about itself. Rather, a caterpillar naturally follows the inner call to withdraw into the silence of its cocoon, it activates dormant components of its DNA, and it emerges as a butterfly to begin life anew.

To be conscious of the Oneness and to connect with the Cosmos from mother Earth is to understand that humanity is part of a living being on a larger scale: Earth, or Lady Gaia. In the same way that interactions occur in our physical bodies among an infinite number of lifeforms: tissues, cells, bacteria — all cohabitating within a single greater being — there is also synergy and interaction between human life and Earth. And beyond Earth, interaction with the galaxy and, even beyond our galaxy, with the universe. Throughout history, humanity has behaved toward Earth the way parasites do: instead of offering healthy benefits to all, they cause illnesses and pains. One way or another, we are like planets ourselves, both on the surface and in our interior, where there are millions of tiny organisms that we call bacteria. Their objective is to contribute to our health and growth, as the bacterial flora of the skin does when it balances our PhD, or the intestinal flora that strengthen our immune system.

Bacteria collaborate with the functioning of our body while participating in a balanced relationship of mutual service and harmony. However, there are also bacteria within the body that forget their initial function and become pathogenic, harmful, eventually becoming a disease. In this case, we find ourselves obliged to eliminate them through our immune system or medication. Of course, for me, this kind of illness or "damage" is also part of our growth process, so that we can evolve and learn in an environment that we created, allowing them to overgrow within us.

As above, so below. In a sense, humans are the equivalent of bacteria on a larger scale. In a state of healthy symbiosis, all life grows as we grow. We all develop as evolving beings, though at times some humans choose to behave in a destructive manner as part of their learning. The dimensional leap involves making the heart vibrate at the same frequency as that of the planet and its new beat, going from egotistic behavior to an awareness of planetary and galactic oneness that makes possible the synergistic coexistence with the new Earth, the Sun, the solar system and the entire Milky Way.

This is the metamorphosis: as humans we coexist with the Earth and awaken to an infinite Consciousness that goes beyond the limits of the planet and the galaxy, recalling how beings live in symbiosis with the environment, nature and all living things.

THIS IS THE TIME for transformation and evolution. Nothing is superfluous, or lacking. Everything is perfect!

Everything fits perfectly, combining in absolute harmony that which is spiritual and physical, inner and outer, material and transcendent, physical and metaphysical, individual and collective, as well as personal and societal. It is understood from the heart that all experiences, regardless of origin or outcome, have a reason for being in the infinite natural process of Love, in which everything flows with the perfection of what Is. Attachments that chain and bind us are released; we become aware that we have always been illuminated, but that this illumination consists, precisely, of realizing that we do not need to be enlightened because we are already light in its various intensities.

IRB allows you, dear reader, to remember your purpose in life, the purpose that led you to incarnate in the current physical life to witness the experiences many lived. They were a part of a new dream that is already behind. It is as if we got out of the pool, and when we dried ourselves off, we saw the whole experience of being in the pool was a dream.

To unify is to stop living a life of individualism, of separation, on the stage of the great theater that is this world. We do this without forgetting that, while we were in the pool we swallowed water and felt like we were drowning, swam in various styles and even snorkeled. Now everything is within you, in your conscience, in your memory, in your DNA, in the experience of being who you are. All this is activated, not to hurt or victimize anyone, but to be of service to the All. Life is like a great collective lesson that helps us move from forgetfulness to consciousness. This allows us to activate the inner child, who cherishes innocence, authenticity, and takes events exactly as they come. It's about understanding the role we play without judging or controlling it, but allowing it to activate the creative capacity that includes all the lessons learned during the scenarios of a chosen incarnation.

To see perfection in each creature that we come across, that is true unity. That is the Oneness expressed by the Sanskrit word *Namaste*.

Being aware that we are consciousness, allows us to see ourselves as we are: Love. It allows us to see God's face, which means recognizing the perfection within every single one of us, and within Everything.

The expression *Namaste*, recognizes, greets, and reveres the Divinity within each being. It stops being a literary expression, an intellectual elaboration, and transforms into a manifestation of absolute unity in which the "I" disappears.

In the state of grace that allows us to genuinely honor and live this manifestation, we become aware that joy is our natural state. Joy doesn't require a specific reason; being happy is an active part of the New Earth and the seed of the new humanity. This new human race that allows all expressions of life, in unison with the metamorphosis of the Earth, ends the martyrdom of duality. In harmony with each person's voluntary progression toward different dimensional scenarios, humanity manifests Heaven on the New Earth. We can access information from the higher dimensions and then make it a reality here in 3D.

It's almost like experiencing resurrection while being alive. Being reborn is not physical, despite the DNA transmutation that are imprinted within each human cell. It is normal to feel lightheadedness and emptiness during this experience because, when we awaken to consciousness, the beliefs that have followed us through the eons cease to be relevant and require a new format. In this new reality, we will experience a very different reality from the one lived during the dream state. The new reality allows us to live in the here and now.

What is difficult to achieve in the dream, becomes natural when living in an awakened state. This characterizes the Love that We Are and that All Is, since here and now is the state in which Love flows and engulfs all that is; the concept of ego dissolves in the Oneness. To achieve this, it is necessary to pulsate from the heart, living in a constant state of surrender, of absolute acceptance, focusing on the inner and mental silence, and forever abandoning intellectual conflicts, which prevent us from living, listening, speaking, thinking, feeling, and acting from the heart.

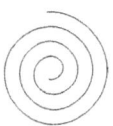

Chapter XII

IRB a Quantum Leap, an Existential Leap

For true love is inexhaustible; the more you give, the more you have.

Antoine de Saint-Exupéry

God, the universe, the Infinite, Universal Mind, Spirit —whatever name you wish to give Source — from a place of Oneness, emanates limitless energy capable of creating changes throughout this planet and its inhabitants. We are at the right moment to be conscious of this.

Earth is going through a cosmic event that generates profound transformations. The energy this generates causes everything to vibrate at higher frequencies, which is why we must be in tune with these vibrations. And just as our world is transforming its limiting energies, we too can transform our current fears into the pure energy of Love; this way, we accept from birth our true nature as super-beings.

The quantum leap causing this change represents the absolute certainty of the end of our dark years and the beginning of the dawn of Living Light for the human race: the Koradi race that will populate the New Earth. This New Earth will be in perfect balance with the Indigo Ray now entering it. Dawn begins when night ends.

As discussed in previous chapters, we are energetic beings vibrating at various frequencies, and we attract into our reality whatever vibrates at that same frequency. When we vibrate at the frequency of love now supported by the planet, we allow the Balancing Indigo Ray into our consciousness, and into each atom of our being, thus resonating at higher and higher levels and becoming aware of the higher dimensions in union with our Creative Source. It is for us to choose to tune into the Indigo Ray Balancing frequency.

IRB energy is capable of changing our molecular structure, mutating our DNA and allowing us to make the leap referred to as the quantum leap or existential leap. A quantum leap occurs when external forces cause an atom to change its structure. In other words, it isn't just about a leap of faith but an existential leap in our DNA. Currently, the base of our DNA is made up of carbon, but IRB frequencies transform it to silicone, which is the crystal base of quartz crystal, the purest transparency that belongs to and brings with it the Koradi race.

The light particles known as photons are what trigger the inner molecular configuration connecting us to the various dimensions of Unity, which allows us to understand that each of our actions affects others. This is one of the main factors that awaken our Wisdom, reminding us of our right to our unlimited and divine ancestral powers.

The consciousness of Oneness, tuned to the frequency of Love, is the quickest path to the great renovation which, in short, consists of being aware that we can create a brand new reality from Oneness. We must raise our vibrations and surrender negative thoughts to the power of infinite Love, infinite Presence, infinite Compassion and infinite Wisdom, and have direct communication with Source, in perfect balance, harmony and absolute neutrality with the Zero Point Field, to believe and create.

If you have reached this point, dear reader, it is a clear sign that you have awakened. Now you must simply tune into the highest frequencies of the planet at this marvelous time you have chosen to live. Balance your entire self with the Indigo Ray that comes from beyond the Pleiades, through the consciousness of the person writing this book, to find joy in each moment of this quantum existence.

As mentioned in Chapter VII, it is individual work with the aim of achieving global transformation through our collective connection. Do you accept this opportunity?

Do you dare to see, feel, imagine, intuit, think and transform your own reality, and that of everyone else, into a world of peace, love and harmony, in perfect balance and creativity? Would you like to be a part of this synchronized planetary orchestration?

If your answer is yes, keep reading. If you would like to go further, listen to the seminar that will activate this information within you in a simple way to make it a reality in your daily life.

Visit us bit.ly/XimenaDuqueValencia_IRB

THIS IS THE TIME FOR TRANSMUTATION.

In experimental science, when we refer to transmutation it is assumed that we mean something esoteric, something separate from Newtonian reality; therefore, this term is typically only be used in philosophy and religion. However, research in electromagnetism and quantum physics has given us reliable tools to question old postulates. Nobel Prize winners in physics and chemistry have conducted extensive research on carbon-12, which is the base of the biological form of all manifestations of nature, and its transmutation under certain circumstances of solar influence. This change is from a 6-6-6 chord to a 6-6-1.

This means transmutation of carbon-12 into carbon-7, an unknown carbon isotope that alters not only the Newtonian field, but the metaphysical as well.

Just as in quantum physics and computer science, we count on great advances that resemble what IRB does for the human computer. Serge Haroche from the Normal Superior School in Paris, and David Wineland from the National Institute of Norms and Technology in Maryland, received the Nobel Peace Prize in 2012 for "directly observing individual quantum particles without destroying them" (Swedish Royal Academy of Sciences).

Haroche developed an efficient method of working with individual atoms. Quantum physics applied to computers is perhaps the easiest way to appreciate this type of work—which will be explained in further detail later—. When finally put into practice, this could mean a revolution even greater than that created by the Internet in recent decades.

While the methodology is well known (the theory has been almost completely developed), the challenge is to overcome the technological barriers. The capacity of machines capable of holding a quantum system with hundreds of thousands of particles must be exponentially greater. In order to be able to simulate quantum processes, a classical computer would have to be gigantic, since its capacity would grow in a linear direction, or linearly, which is how we have been told to think throughout human history, linearly, even though the mind is an entirely quantum system.

Richard Feynman was the first to raise this critique of classical computational physics by proposing the use of a simple quantum unit called the qubit (quantum bit), as the basic structural element of a new computer. That is how the dream of a quantum computer was born, a machine much more advanced than today's classical computer, which functions based on a binary system of ones and zeros.

The quantum computer functions with the qubit, a combination of zeros and ones that can transfigure themselves in different ways, generating more possibilities for storing data. Meaning, it can be simultaneously in two different states. Possibilities continuously range between zero and one, with overlays containing more or less than the two classical states, zeros and ones, all at once. If we describe the qubit in terms of a vector, we could say that the length of this vector is fixed but capable of pointing in any direction — unlike the classical bit, which can only point up or down. This is precisely the point of quantum physics: that reality can be understood in other ways. For example, we see a person going up or down the hill; in quantum physics this person can go both up and down at the same time, and this is referred to as a dichotomous situation.

Thus, speaking in quantum terms, an object can be two different things at the same time, just so long as they are opposites, such as going up or down. The linear time in which we have lived in the 3D world is completely limiting; conversely, the multi-dimensional permits us to see that past, present and future occur within the same space and time in different dimensions. If computers were programmed in superposed ones and zeros simultaneously, in practical terms it would be like putting together hundreds of thousands of computers to work together as one. Complicated tasks could be done in microseconds, creating infinite possibilities that we never even imagined, in infinitesimal time spans.

The above explanation is to illustrate briefly how IRB puts human beings in a quantum state. It's something similar to the difference between normal light and laser light; we go from being a light being to being a Living Light in action.

Let's talk about the importance of the number 13 in IRB. The number 13 was very significant in Mayan philosophy. It represented the thirteen principles that make up the seven laws of creation; Mayans gave very particular connotations to the number 13, such as 12+1, where 12 represents the number of the Temple, meaning the physical, that which houses the spirit, while the 1 represents the spirit. For example, many monuments have twelve columns plus one altar. Its more exact meaning is that mass manifests up to the number 12, such as the twelve helixes of our DNA (our genetic code), and the "+1 factor" references the spiritual, the 1 being eternal Unity.

Because of the significance of the unification of the material and spiritual planes, it is necessary to transform the manipulation we were subjected to, using the 12:60 matrix (i.e., the Gregorian calendar and the clock) and everything related to the 12 frequency. Why? Because it restricts us by creating identification with matter. When we recognize the frequency of 13, we identify with a higher vibration of being. The number 13 is the subtleness of the spirit that nonetheless prevails over the material.

In other fields such as Tibetan Theosophy and sacred geometry, we find concepts such as the thirteen modules of RAM memory of the soul. The 6-6-1 was mentioned earlier (the C-7 isotope adds up to thirteen). It is also said that one grand cycle of rotation of our planet is 5,125 years; these numbers also add up to thirteen.

There are many myths surrounding the number 13, such as being a bringer of bad luck, thus we take special care on the thirteenth of the month; some hotels don't include a thirteenth floor in their design, and many elevators ignore it. Certain airplanes do not have a thirteenth row; Madrid's metro system does not use that number, and countless other examples prove that the manipulators are hiding from us these symbols of great power.

Yet we see this sacred number included in the sacred geometry of the Fibonacci series, and camouflaged in many symbols used by the Power Elite.

There are thirteen moons in a year, as shown by the Mayan, Hebrew and Chinese calendars, and all the other calendars that count days in a natural way rather than a synthetic way like the Gregorian calendar, which is very far removed from the natural flow of cosmic movements. The Knights of King Arthur were twelve, and he was the thirteenth Knight. Traditional Chinese medicine works with thirteen meridians mapped throughout our bodies, and musicians use a scale composed of thirteen notes, including sustained notes.

The most impressive manifestation of the power of the number 13 is revealed within a carbon isotope that was unknown until very recently: carbon-7. There are a considerable number of articles regarding the 2012 discovery of rays being emitted from the sun that disintegrate radioactive elements on earth — causative of the mutation of matter, and influential in the speed of the decay of elements like carbon-14. This phenomenon has become a subject of scientific study. Carbon is the base of life as we know it on our planet, and carbon-12 is the most abundant, representing approximately 99% of all known carbon. It is a carbon isotope that contains six protons, six neutrons, and six electrons, 6-6-6.

Carbon-12 is the second most important element in the human body, right after oxygen. And, following hydrogen, helium, and oxygen, it is the fourth most abundant element in the universe. Carbon-12 is also one of the five elements that compose human DNA, making it one of the most important components in the manifestation of life in this dimension. We could interpret this as being what John, author of the book of Revelations, sometimes referred to as "the Apocalypse of John." He wrote that 666 was the number of man, or the number of the beast, because that's what connects us to the material, the physical base of the human body, and what confines us to the physical universe.

If we are able to transmute carbon-12, we can obtain — or rather, recover — superhuman powers, which would make all today's technological advances obsolete. Regardless of how important they were to our progress up to this point, they would simply be a mirror that shows us what we can do for ourselves without depending on any type of physical apparatus, since all information is available within the totality.

All secrets have their time of disclosure, and this may be the biggest of our time: activating our alchemical powers. Not the old-fashioned alchemy that attempted to transform lead into gold. That was a metaphoric way to understand and access our undreamed-of higher dimensions.

Carbon-7 is the carbon isotope that has six electrons, six protons and only one neutron, a relation also present in the kundalini system, represented by masculine and feminine opposites: — six inferior energetic centers in the human body and a seventh neutral center referred to as sahasraara in Sanskrit. That is a connector to Zero Point, like in Metatron's Cube, which is constructed from a central circle surrounded by six spheres, then six more on the outside, which composes 6-6-1, or 12+1. (In Judaism, Metatron is considered the mediator between God and man.)

The aforementioned cube reminds us that sacred geometry evolved from the merkabah (field of light) explained in depth and in a fascinating way by the most controversial quantum physicist of our time, Nassim Haramein. He, a Swiss man of Middle Eastern origin, explained the creation of the universe with a tetrahedron. Just as a magnet is able to maintain a magnetic field around it, carbon-7 has the ability to maintain hyper-dimensional fields — such as thought — around it in amplified and unlimited ways.

When looking at images of saints and other enlightened beings, what we may see as a gold aura or halo of light around their heads, is in fact the luminosity of neutrons due to the high amount of carbon-12 being transformed into carbon-7 in their brains. That gives them powers that we would call supernatural, but in reality those powers could become part of our daily lives if we recognized the Original model of perfection as a part of each of us. This carbon-7 quickly changes to other forms of more stable mass, thus it is impossible to directly detect in the human body.

This piece of knowledge has been hidden for centuries, one that cannot be uncovered with the intellect but through consciousness; however, it has begun to come to light, perhaps because we are ready to take this quantum leap, or simply because when going from Galactic winter to Galactic spring, the light allows us to see what was present but undetectable due to the prevailing darkness.

The Light shines brightly now, and now we can see that which has been there all along. This allows for the most important evolution humanity has ever gone through: transforming fear into Love. THIS IS THE TIME for all secrets to be revealed.

In Christian lore, The Last Supper, a scene painted by many artists including Leonardo Da Vinci, illustrates a moment before the crucifixion of Christ. It is another symbolic representation of the 6-6-1 configuration: six apostles on either side of the Master.

It is interesting to observe that kundalini, Metatron, and Christ are all vessels of ascension, despite their being in different spiritual systems. They are the Zero Point, the number 13.

This knowledge is understood by beings of the highest spheres, perhaps inhabitants of other dimensions, planets or galaxies. It becomes visible and accessible as information through the intention of expanding the mind to create the consciousness of Oneness.

Obviously this is a gradual metamorphosis, not an instant mutation. (It is estimated that the change will be complete in the year 2018 of this new era.) The human being requires a period of adjustment in which the collective mind is subjected to quantum expansion. A critical mass in humanity must go from the egocentric material life to a life were ego does not dominate, vibrating in the frequency of Love. The Sun's activity during this time is heightened, and the final transmutation be balancing the Indigo Ray, producing the transformation in human DNA of carbon-12 into carbon-7. This gives the human being power to migrate to the New Earth and access information found in superior dimensions; it is a synchronization of un-time, which cannot be understood by the intellect but only through the totality of the Self.

The planet's vibration is continuously rising, which has repercussions on the vibrations of every manifestation of life on the surface and within. The evolution of the physical body from carbon form to crystal form is based on the carbon atom, which is unchangeable. What IRB reflects is a change in the configuration of the cell, which continues to accelerate. The connection between the left and right hemispheres of the brain also increases, and this contributes in part to awakening, since "the intuitive I" becomes more active.

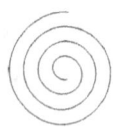

Chapter XIII
Your Choice

So long as we practice these in our daily lives, then no matter if we are learned or unlearned, whether we believe in Buddha or God, or follow some other religion, or none at all; as long as we have compassion for others and conduct ourselves with restraint from a sense of responsibility, there is no doubt we will be happy..

Dalai Lama

This is only the beginning; a new cycle of 25,625 years is starting. You, me, all of us, are part of the momentum activating this earthly project of Light. Each of us has a mission we must accomplish to contribute to this change in eras. When we express our consciousness at higher vibrational levels, our reality will access superior dimensions and nothing that occurs in the 3D world can affect us. We must focus on tuning into the correct frequency; this is our main objective.

THIS IS THE TIME to awaken and understand that we are unlimited beings; we are Living Light in action. We have chosen to be in this moment in 3D to trigger a transformation and to maximize awareness of being One with consciousness, that of the cosmos, and that of other beings in the vast universe.

It is necessary to understand that our current lives are nothing more than an illusion created by our ego, and that ego only identifies with the personality of the character we are portraying in this play called Life. Let us cast aside the role that we have been playing and discover our true essence.

IRB tunes us into the highest frequencies of Love and thus allows us to change the frequencies of fear into Love. The great and powerful groups of religions, politics and economics, have tried to keep us from discovering Love. We must, however, be grateful to them since they too are part of this grand process. The key is to let go of any information that might lower our vibratory frequency to the level of fear. And it is important to understand that said groups have blinded our eyes by creating opposites that are actually "opposimilar;" they have us believing that we have the ability to choose when what we are actually doing is killing ourselves defending their choices. This is part of the game where there are always losers and winners; this is why the only way for the game to end, is not to oppose it or look for a formula to win it, but to simply stop taking part.

Let us access the sixty-four initial codes that make up the foundation of our DNA with its active thirteenth Layer. Love is a very high frequency with a very short wavelength, which means there are more points of contact in our DNA when we vibrate at this frequency. They are all controlled by four nuclear commands that have always been there and are now visible and possible to activate through IRB. The more points of contact that we awaken, the more genetic codes we activate. THIS IS THE TIME to permanently awake in a new reality, a world of peace, love and harmony among all human beings and all manifestations of life.

Let us remember that exterior reality is a reflection of internal reality. If we find peace, love, and harmony within, our outer world will vibrate at the same frequency. This is achieved when we balance the Indigo Ray in the body and mind in absolute coherence with the thirteenth Layer of our DNA, which is the director of its own orchestra, a quantum orchestrator.

Awaken to your spiritual reality, dear reader, and be fully conscious that, among other things, you are the creator of your reality through your emotions, your thoughts, your words and your actions. In short, you possess the power to create whatever you wish. You have had this power always. The difference with IRB is that, by permanently tuning into the frequency of Love and transmuting your atoms to C-7 and activating the thirteenth Layer of your DNA to its full potential, you will no longer have to struggle against polarization but simply access it as part of the same formula. No more structures of division and fear!

THIS IS THE TIME TO CHOOSE WISELY, THIS IS THE TIME TO CHOOSE IRB

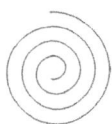

Second Part

Conventional

Chapter XIV
Everything is Energy

Energy cannot be created or destroyed; it can only be changed from one form to another.

Albert Einstein

Lee Carroll, the original channeler of Kryon, was the first to say that 95% of our DNA (which science has called fill-in DNA) is composed of quantum DNA. From that point, many scientists and researchers have come to similar conclusions, to the point of supporting a theory that we are divine quantum beings, and that we have many more abilities and potentials than believed based on our old system of beliefs.

IRB goes along with this theory, delving deeper into the twelve layers of the DNA that Kryon explains through Lee Carroll in his book Kryon XII: The Twelve Layers of DNA, which, along with the importance of the number 13 and the existential leap caused by this vibration, is precisely what activates the Thirteenth Layer, as was explained in the previous chapter.

Believing for so many years that we are only five or ten percent of what we really are, has caused us to also believe in illness, poverty and karma, as has been taught throughout various eras. Medicine and psychology have been seen as playing an important role in fighting diseases and other imbalances. Historically, we have always depended on pharmaceuticals and invasive procedures to heal our physical ailments. Pharmaceuticals, however, only treat our symptoms and generally do not reach the origin of the problem, while continuing to harm our bodies, producing serious side- effects; in cancer, for example, cells are destroyed through radiation or chemotherapy. Cancerous cells, though, are metabolized, just as are the rest of the cells in the body, and learn to defend themselves from chemotherapy and radiation, which makes them more resistant.

What these types of invasive treatments do is deteriorate the DNA of the cells that divide rapidly, but the best way to control a cancerous cell is to augment the power of the cells of the immune system. Unfortunately, the immunized cells divide even more rapidly and so are the first ones affected, destroying the only thing that might save our lives.

Thomas Alva Edison said that doctors of the future would not heal illnesses but rather prevent them through intelligent and healthy nutrition. When we say nutrition, we are not just talking about physical nutrition, what goes through our mouths to give energy to our physical body. The more natural, fresh, organic and raw something is, the longer and more vital the results, allowing us to be more fully present. However, we must also consider emotional nutrition, which is what satisfies our states of mind with permanent feelings of joy and love, with no room for feelings produced by the ego, which are the main contributors to stress in modern life.

Mental nutrition is also essential, since our beliefs are the main contributors to our behavior, which in turn generates the results produced by the emotions. Mental nutrition includes reading, watching movies, going to workshops, surrounding ourselves with inspiring people, and optimizing the information that our minds receive, with productive content conducive to constant personal growth, guaranteeing a life of permanent inspiration and creativity while generating thoughts from Wisdom. Here we do not include the media or anything that may contradict the truth that we are unlimited beings. To remain spiritually fed, connected to Source, in service, in acceptance, and in consciousness, is to experience Compassion at its fullest, with the profound understanding that We Are One.

The lack of good nutrition, in every sense, makes the organism vulnerable to the free radicals inside it, producing aging, illness and death. This is why it is of vital importance to keep our immune system in optimal condition; it is our greatest ally in keeping any type of illness or unbalance at bay. We remain alert when the central nervous system is kept healthy, without stress to destabilize it.

In short, it doesn't matter the symptom or the illness, what is important is to reestablish the energy and information of the Original Model to create states of health and abundance, results that, based on our current beliefs, would not be possible. Reestablishing the origin of our quantum DNA and all its power, activating all the current information, is what IRB is about.

To try to obtain information anchored in cellular memory through lived experiences worsens the imbalance, since it opens old wounds that the organism once tried to heal. To prescribe painkillers or antibiotics to eliminate infection or viruses is continuing to contribute to the cells closing to conserve the energy of the body and thus limiting oxygen, nutrients, and glucose — fuel for the cells — from entering the cell, causing the mitochondria, which have a very similar composition to bacteria, to not be nourished. The same things that happen to the mitochondria, happen to the cells, and happen to the body.

A great part of the manipulation that we discussed at the beginning of the book, comes from the pharmaceutical industry, which will have us believing that by alleviating symptoms, we heal ourselves. In reality the only result is that this industry makes more money, as well as anchoring strong beliefs into humanity about their dependency on drugs. Instead, when we speak of healing through energy, frequencies, information, quantum physics, the power of thought, and spirituality, we are talking about very serious subjects, among them the elimination of old paradigms at a global level. To learn more about this, there is no better way than to read David Icke.

Energy exists within everything. Light, for example, is a frequency of energy that we detect with our eyes; sound is a frequency or vibration that we perceive with our ears, with our feet and with our skin; infrared energy is detected as heat or as ultraviolet light and is found beyond what we can see within the spectrum of light. There are many other frequencies of energy that exist for which we do not have active receptors in our body at this moment, such as x-rays, ultrasound, radar, UHF, VHF, and many more. Since we cannot detect them with our physical senses, at some point in human history they were considered mystical. However, since science has created instruments that allow us to detect them, we are now aware of their existence, including the ability to send hundreds of thousands of messages every second through a very thin fiber that uses light frequency; though we do not completely understand how the optical fiber works, I am sure that we all use it.

The same thing occurs with our health. Through the highest frequencies that have yet to be detected by scientific equipment in our 3D, we have been able to eradicate an unlimited number of bodily and mental imbalances. And now the whole of the Indigo Ray is here to activate deep Balance in the entirety of the self, through INDIGO RAY BALANCING, or IRB.

It takes years, even centuries, for an old belief to be completely eradicated from collective consciousness, even when it is not interacted with. Fortunately, more and more people are beginning to understand energy as quantum physics describes it, despite this being ignored by general education.

Generally, pioneers who wish to change old theories tend to be misunderstood and sometimes persecuted and judged. In the first part of this book, we talked about how Copernicus dared to state that both planet Earth and other known planets turned around the Sun. Later Galileo mathematically proved Copernicus's theory. Then Christopher Columbus, in his rush to confirm that the world was round, "discovered" the American continent. Many others tried to seek the truth through science and were persecuted.

Human beings tend to get attached to theories out of fear of change, being different, breaking paradigms, being judged, though many times the old theories end up not being true, since many times they were established to manipulate and pigeonhole norms and behaviors that would prevent the discovery of truth. Only when we dare to create our own ways of being and thinking will we be close to our true being, understanding revelations as healthy, since our Original Model is perfect. Only the truth will set us free; keeping ourselves in ignorance is to surrender our future to others, which is up to us in the present moment.

We have seen quantum physics explain the way the universe works, and the understanding of this theory has led to great discoveries in health. Therefore, "healing" many illnesses, as Lynne McTaggart points out in The Field (2006), a book documenting the findings of quantum physics experiments in medicine, as part of the new understanding, means a change of thought. Physics have not been modified, it has simply changed along with our way of understanding and applying it, and there will probably be more surprises, as evolution does not stop. The truth never changes; what changes is our way of perceiving.

To be able to balance this energy, to shape it as we see fit while including and recognizing physical, mental, emotional and spiritual perfection, and other areas that we cannot even begin to imagine, is what IRB offers us.

What's important is to synchronize natural processes from the totality of our being in such a way as to attune ourselves to the truth that stops old age and reverses any process of disease, whatever it may be. This is achieved by going directly to the cause in the DNA and not the symptoms. Incorporating the knowledge we have gained from our experiences, accessing the Zero Point Field in the layers of our DNA, using the frequencies of healthy energy in the organism, without ignoring destructive frequencies, which are opposites, is key.

Just as light brightens the darkness, healthy energy, the Original Model in the divine being, regenerates dissolute energy; even better, it connects us to the supreme essence where destructive frequencies are not present. With healthy frequencies, neutrality creates a new reality. Thus we can coexist with respect and balance with everything that is; that means no war, and therefore no winners or losers. Game over.

All that which we call problems, lack, or disease, are only imbalances in the dimension that we have chosen as a learning ground. They have been part of our learning and life's journey, presented as challenges in our health, our relationships, our professional environments, our performance, and everything we can imagine. All of this is related to the energetic balance in the body and the frequency to which we resonate. Therefore, understanding our history and our heritage, learning to think with the heart and feel with the mind, is of great help. And yet, for this to stand the test of time, we must activate the totality of our quantum DNA, including the Thirteenth Layer. This is the true secret.

The complete information exists in the field. The critical factor is our transference of the information into 3D where we believe ourselves to be linear.

To illustrate this, let us refer to chemicals that pass from molecule to molecule in a rhythm that is almost one centimeter per second, and very few are lost in each transference — while the transference of information through frequencies occurs at almost 300,000 km/s, meanwhile losing practically none of it. This is why cell phones and the Internet have become such useful tools in our days, since they allow almost instantaneous communication, which thirty years ago would have been a sci-fi fantasy such as Star Trek. The frequencies allow for the totality of our being to adjust, and IRB makes it possible for our DNA to return to the divine Original Model of Adam Kadmon, of our pure and perfect essence, making this transference from levels of Living Light and Love.

Let us again use the Internet as an example. We can say that the information is on the web, and the internet is the Spirit, the field, the Source, or whatever we want to call it. The human body is the hardware where the software is installed, which is shaped by our thoughts and emotions. The frequencies are the connection, the bandwidth that connects to the web, and IRB is the interface that allows everything to become useful and practical. The information can be used at the right moment from any of the existing dimensions of the web. From Love, Presence, Compassion and Wisdom, it can be used in any area that is required in the life mission of each person.

The beginning of any imbalance is learned information, information that has been coded into our DNA; therefore, all healing occurs when we change this information from the root of the DNA, or better yet when we incorporate the learning that is offered by this information into our field, into our genetic history. To access this root, or the Zero Point Field, that connects us to the dimension in which we have learned, it is important to eliminate the stress that keeps us from accessing the most profound truths. When we are able to eliminate stress, everything in our life begins to again find balance and divine order, in accord with our Original Model. When we return to our Divine Human Being, everything can be healed or, better stated: disease and unbalance do not exist.

Research done by the University of Stanford and the HeartMath Institute in California indicates that if we could eliminate stress, we could permanently heal even genetic problems. Meaning, not only would we heal on our own, but we would heal future generations. And when we heal our quantum DNA, we also heal future lives.

For many years science believed that all memories were stored in the brain, and in the search for that specific place, scientists cut into each part of the brain, discovering that the majority of memories were not stored in the brain. Memories are stored directly to our DNA, which is in the totality of our body. Our cells are our "hard drive," and we know very well that information stored in a hard drive is susceptible to being modified. When that happens, the computer's behavior also changes.

Great scientists such as doctors Howard, Antonio Damasio, chief of the Department of neurology in the University of South California, and Lipton, jointly affirm that cellular memories are stored in our cells; not only in the cells of the brain but in the entire body. They all maintain that memory is made up of images, which means that each thought generated is associated with an image, which in turn means that we are some sort of photographic camera that archives everything in its databank: the cells. And once an image is generated, our emotions categorize them as good, bad, anxious or traumatizing, which our belief system reinforces with the software of anger, bitterness, resentment, fear — or the opposite: joy, gratitude, love, satisfaction or pleasure. That is why one of the fundamental objectives of IRB is to change our beliefs, directly from the heart.

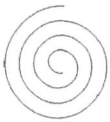

Chapter XV
Cellular Memory

To repress emotions and not let them flow freely is to set up a dis-integrity in the system, causing it to act at cross-purposes rather than as a unified whole. The stress this creates, which takes the form of blockages and insufficient flow of peptide signals to maintain function at the cellular level, is what sets up the weakened conditions that can lead to disease.

Candace Pert
Neuroscientist and Pharmacologist

There are many documented cases of people who have received organ transplants having thoughts, feelings, dreams, and even the personality and personal tastes of the donors. Now many scientists are convinced that such memories are stored in cells in the entire body and not just in one specific place.

Southwestern University published a study in 2004 that stated, "The cell memories are like little Post-it notes that tell the cell what to do—only when there are destructive cell memories, the Post-its are telling the cell to do the wrong thing."

IRB allows for the download of new information that contains the Original Model of the divine code created from the transmission of Living Light and Love into our bodies and minds, allowing us to access this dimension of living in total balance.

When we do not experience conscious living, it is the ego that filters the information transmitted to our cells, and that type of information creates imbalance, anxiety, stress, and the limiting beliefs that initiate the stress response in the body. These limiting beliefs attach themselves to our cellular memory, which is what informs the conscious and subconscious minds, along with the control centers of the brain.

The HeartMath Institute has put emphasis on alternative research of what was once thought unbelievable but has since turned out to be true. Among these experiments, one in particular caught my attention. It had a lot to do with the experiments of Dr. Masaru Emoto in regard to changing the morphology of water, except this time the clinic experimented directly with DNA. The scientists put human DNA in a test tube then instructed people to hold it in their hands while thinking about painful situations, destructive events, or what we would call "tough lessons." We all know it is possible to have painful feelings just remembering destructive events.

After this, the researchers took the DNA from the test tube and examined it, finding the DNA damaged. Then they took the same DNA, placed it in another test tube and asked people to hold it in their hands while thinking good or happy thoughts (we can access these feelings because they are stored in our cellular memory). Then they took the DNA out of the test tube, examined it and discovered that there had been a healing effect on the previously damaged DNA.

This indicates that the activation of certain memories is capable of altering our DNA, whereas the activation of healthy memories can reconstruct or return to its original state DNA previously affected by old patterns of thought. Therefore, it is not enough to think positively in the now, but also to perceive events in a positive way, as a single fluid process from Love, so that we can, through an

Cellular Memory

evolutionary change of consciousness, reform it into the Original Model without distortion.

For this to happen, it is necessary to have access to the totality of the DNA, including that which science has deemed for years "junk DNA," which are actually our quantum or divine layers, based on the information that Kryon gave Carroll (2010) in The Twelve Layers of DNA: An Esoteric Study of the Mastery Within. According to Rochev Baaravot, memory is anchored in the Eighth Layer of our DNA.

It has been proven that chronic pain and other illnesses stem from feelings triggered by fear, such as anger and many other destructive emotions repressed in the subconscious mind; meaning, we are not consciously aware of these feelings that we carry inside, let alone that we have been storing them for eons. Anger is rooted in our cellular memory. Given that We Are All One, whatever each of us thinks, says, feels and does, affects the rest. And if we are able to affect the entire community through the collective subconscious or the critical mass, imagine how a parent's worry can directly influence the illness or pain of a child. In other words, the parents' stress creates limiting cellular memories that end up manifesting as pain, illness and limiting behaviors in their children. This is why when we heal our DNA of limiting beliefs, we are healing our quantum experience and that of future generations.

Many known healing systems can cure many of the afflictions generated by cellular memories, but after a while they may resurface and we relapse into physical, mental or emotional imbalance. Our responsibility in the new energy invites us to achieve long-term healing, permanently, if we rid ourselves of memories and feelings of anger, sadness, fear, confusion, guilt, impotence and an endless list of other limiting emotions, instead making the decision to have positive thoughts. We must strive to lose identification with form, to remain unchanged and unmoved in each present moment, to activate our consciousness by transforming the ego in the eternal present. We must become conscious — from a perspective of learning and Love — of everything contained in our cellular memory, within our DNA, not only of this present earthly existence but also our Aathmic imprint.

IRB exists so we do not have to "heal." That is the first paradigm that it has to shatter: we do not need to heal; we simply need to tune into the dimension where we already live in perfect health. Viewing this idea from a different perspective, history is not erased; it is rewritten.

Psychology for example, has tried to find a way to cure cellular memories, though in many cases speaking of problems over and over tends to worsen them.

Neurolinguistic Programming (NLP) can train us to think differently about success, allowing us to reframe it, which is a great help because it eliminates suffering and pain. Additionally, NLP explains why, of all memories of anything that has ever happened to us, more than 90% are stored in our conscious or unconscious. This means that it is very difficult, and almost impossible, to remember them. Meaning that only about 10% of our memories are conscious and we can change them if we try. To illustrate this point, we can use the metaphor of an iceberg: 90% of our memories are beneath water level, and only 10% float above it.

The aforementioned only refers to this current existence, the one we are clearly conscious of. But if the memory originates in a life in another existence or another dimension, then it is archived in the Eighth Layer of our DNA, where we find the accumulation of all experiences lived in past lives, parallel lives — ourselves in other realities or dimensions — and future lives. It is in our DNA that we find our unconscious mind, our consciousness, and our spiritual imprint. This is the totality of what we are, including our human genome, our emotions, our ascension vehicle, our Jacob's ladder, our I Am, our self-mastery, our divine mark, our perfection, our creative self and our Divinity. The sum of all of the information in the universe is in each of our cells, which connect to the DNA of all that is, of Source, of the divine essence, that which allows us to return to our original state. It allows us to return to our origin, to Paradise, to what we have called Eden. IRB makes this an easy and beautiful path.

While traditional medicine balances the chemicals in our brain, the chemical discrepancy is a symptom of learning and so can't be directly healed in this way. This is what we have realized through the years: if we cure the symptoms, the imbalance continues; thus we have only learned ways to manage pain. What we truly want is to restore Balance to our lives forever, in this life and in any existence on any plane that we decide to experience.

This is why IRB focuses on exchanging the pattern of energy in the destructive cellular memory for the Divine Original Model. IRB's goal is to change forever the face of health. When we say health, we are referring to everything that surrounds a person on a daily basis. We hope to stabilize the inner frequencies that generate imbalances in the body by accessing information from the highest levels. This information increases the vibration of the mind and body of each person or being on the planet, transforming the body's energy pattern.

We have a way to archive images and memories with the software of our choice; that is why it is very important to change our inner perception of things, so that the photo or film is sustained by beneficial emotions, instead of those that make us sick and limit us. Therefore, it is important to reprogram ourselves from the heart, not from the brain, so that, when we change our consciousness from the nucleus of our cells, we can generate a new film that empowers our divine capacity.

Experiences can become beliefs, and these can be either empowering or destructive and limiting. All of them, whatever type they are, lead to the activation of imbalance in the body, the disconnection of the immune system, and various problems in our lives. The substance of memories and images is a range of energy frequencies, which are also the language of the heart, determining our behavior. When we give free reign to painful or sad memories of depression or anger, and we allow our focus to turn to them, we give free reign to negative emotions, eventually causing our organism to have patterns of disease.

We can consciously choose good and healthy memories and thoughts, but the subconscious 90% beneath the iceberg is impossible to re-direct, for the subconscious chooses what to think, as it works by association. This means that when you are in a negative situation similar to one lived in the past, the subconscious mind reactivates those negative thoughts and we begin to feel bad without knowing why. This happens all the time and causes problems in our lives, which is why it is important to download the new information to the DNA of our cells.

Lipton (2005) in The Biology of Belief confirms that a mistaken belief can cause us to be fearful when we should not be. This explains why sometimes we ask ourselves things like: why am I angry when there is no reason to be? Why do I eat so much even though I know I shouldn't? Why do I think about things that I don't actually want to think about? Why is it that, if I want to think about good, healthy, positive things, I can't seem to shake off the situation that triggers other thoughts, feelings and behavior? Because the situation is nested in the nucleus of the cells and not in the brain; that is why it is so important to change the program, the perspective in the way we remember. Not unlike a computer, we must completely decode and replace the system to get rid of any virus or malicious software that can limit future programs of a different kind.

Besides carrying the memories stored in this life, we are also marked by past, parallel and future lives, because everything in quantum time is the same "soup," inseparable and indivisible. But to be able to live this human experience, we need the vessels of a mother and a father, who carry the imprint of their own lives. This means that we not only store our own complications, but also those of our parents, who for their part carry their own issues, and that of our grandparents, and thus grows the pyramid, storing an infinite amount of information from all our ancestors. What we must truly "heal" is the point of the pyramid, the origin. When we bring Balance to Everything, identity stops being about the person or the event, since we then understand that we are the process itself, the event itself, the Presence and perfection.

To be aware of a person's thoughts, beliefs and behavior can stem from something that did not even happen in their lives. This can be quite frustrating and lead to desperation, hopelessness and illness. This is one of the reasons why traditional healing techniques have not been effective for a great percentage of people throughout history. It is very complicated to treat a problem that we do not even know exists. But if we simply introduce new information to the cell, in the totality and infinite Wisdom appertaining to its own quantum DNA, we are coming from origin, regardless of what has been before, or how much erroneous or limiting information there is within it, since now it is all incorporated as lessons from Love.

The most powerful and surprising thing is not so much that we are able to heal the individual, but that we can also heal the society that gave birth to it, entire races — from the individual to the world, without limits! By returning the person to their Original Model, IRB reestablishes order, not only in the person, but in the society to which they belong, since everything is connected.

In our childhoods, we learned by way of memory. The level of reasoning at the moment we live an experience equals the level of consciousness of an infant that does not possess all of the information, but only that of his little world. For this reason, experiences lived in our early years are embedded in our cellular memory, without going through the filter of conscious judgment. For example, if a baby cries hungrily at midnight, or has a wet diaper, and the response is an angry mother or a father who sees to it only grudgingly, the baby cannot understand that his parents worked arduously all day and need their rest. The baby's experience only absorbs the reality that in his desire to avoid discomfort like hunger or wet diapers, he has to face parents who, at that moment, are not very loving.

This creates confusion, and in his adult life this cellular memory can resurface when the time comes to satisfy physical needs, seek the love of another, or even each time he or she wakes up in the middle of the night. This is only a small example of how the variety of memories, fears and pains stored in each second of our lives can, in the end, block our health, well-being, relationships, success at work, interpersonal relationships, our sense of worth, abundance and numerous aspects of daily life.

Every time these memories are reactivated, we revert to the same young age we were when they were recorded, not as adults who can experience them in a rational way, because what triggers them is the reactive mind and not the logical one.

Can we change what has already been lived? Can we go back in time? Can we dig deep into our files and rationalize each memory so that we can heal it? No. But we can access new information that allows us to observe it and feel it in a different way at the nucleus of the cell, transforming not only the memories but the complete history of our DNA.

Just as the foot reacts without using logic and steps on the brake pedal when the vehicle in front makes a sudden stop, in the same way, our DNA violently reacts to stimulation stored in the DNA. This is what Dr. Lipton means when he says that people are afraid when they should not be. Fear keeps us from acting in the positive way we are able to; it does not allow us to relate to love the way we wish to; it closes our cells, and we have already seen what it is like when cells are closed, how they are not nourished, and when they are not nourished, illness results.

This is the main reason why we so often say or do things that go against what we truly want in our lives, without knowing why. If we don't remove these memories from the learning process, they become belief systems that pretend to protect us, and the same beliefs proceed to our conscious mind, which then tunes us into duality and limits, causing our relationships to end, tasks to not get done, and for us go into victimhood. These memories are stored in the nucleus of our cells and our DNA, which does not differentiate these events as happening in the past; they are happening right now because absolutely everything is present.

Our DNA is at all times living in actual reality, in 360° surround-sound. That is why, when a memory of pain or pleasure is activated, not only are we dealing with something that happened ten, twenty or thirty years ago, or in another lifetime, but also an emergency happening right now. It is at that moment that we react in a state of confusion and conflict. What is felt is very strong and requires our attention. The problem lies in that, at that precise moment, it doesn't make any sense. That is why IRB comes with a new energy of Balance and the power of the Indigo Ray, to live life in love, joy and peace.

Beliefs are an operative system programmed to protect us from repeating painful situations in our lives. Beliefs tend to have an enormous effect in the way we live because they are based on logical reasoning. When the memories of past traumas surface, the rational brain is overridden and the emotional, reactive brain answers the pain, generating stress and latent imbalances. Perhaps the rational brain, merely reacting, makes the decision to disconnect or diminish contact.

My questions to you as you read this book are: are you living the life that you want, or do you find yourself in constant state of confusion? Is it possible for old memories or traumas to be reactivating due to your current circumstances? If your answer is yes, it is the result of painful memories of this life, or past, parallel or future lives, anchored into your DNA. These now have priority over any other type of memory, allowing you to survive and grow.

The bigger the trauma suffered in the past, the greater the probability of its reactivation by any number of associations. Any situation similar to the grievous event will activate it, creating a state of alertness. If this event happened again, we think, we might not be able to survive it this time. This association could be as insignificant as the color of a garment that happened to be nearby when the trauma occurred; everything is anchored in the subconscious.

This makes it so that we don't even know what is happening or why we are feeling what we are feeling, or why we are doing what we are doing. Nevertheless, the only proper way to react is by transforming the information of the hidden memories. To remember may be too painful most of the time, or maybe we do not remember because it is toward the bottom of the iceberg. We might re-experience the pain so intensely that we would re-anchor it, now with new memories and associations. We deserve to learn, change and transcend without the pain, the lack, and the illness. We must recuperate the frequency and the original information of our sacred, quantum DNA for a permanent solution.

To complete the perfection of our cellular system, these memories of trauma are protected by our unconscious mind with the aim

Cellular Memory

of preventing them from being healed. It sounds a bit absurd that, if we become aware of the trauma, our unconscious mind would not want to heal it. But the principle is so simple. The unconscious mind resists the healing of these types of memory as a way of safeguarding itself from similar hurts. It means that if the memory is eliminated, we could once again attract the same experience, and it could be so painful that if we allow it to happen again we might not survive, leading to extremes such as suicide or developing a terrible illness. This is why it is of vital importance to activate the learning that the experience generated from Love, instead of erasing it, so as to not have to repeat it ever again. This is not accomplished through neural reprogramming, or in the brain, or through logic, or anything that uses the will to change the symptoms. It is necessary to go to the origin, the Source, and there is only one origin: DNA.

Many healing techniques that claim to erase things that happened in our past lives, leaving our DNA blank, run the high risk of re-anchoring patterns that we had already overcome. Therefore, the solution is not to erase but to transform the memories with new information that incorporates the lessons of what has already been lived. It is not practical to use the ego to change information, since the ego is always intimately linked to our beliefs, and we always think our beliefs are better because of the patterns we are trying to establish. Only the universal intelligence of Everything can do this transformation. It is the energy of Love and freedom that can clear any type of belief that might once again anchor limiting information codes to future lives from this present.

Chapter XVI

The Power of Belief

Believe nothing, no matter where you read it or who said it, no matter if I have said it, unless it agrees with your own reason and your own common sense.

Buda

There's a story of a math teacher who gave her students a problem to solve, announcing that if they were able to solve it, they would get a special reward, as no one in her class had been able to solve it before. The day she made the announcement, however, one girl was absent and therefore did not hear that the problem was supposed to be unsolvable; due to this, she was the only student to arrive the next day with the problem solved. The wise math teacher understood that, even though the girl was intelligent, she had been able to solve the seemingly impossible problem simply because, without a doubt in her heart, she believed that she could. Solving the math problem was simply the physical manifestation of her inner belief.

What are some "math problems" you currently have in your life? Whatever they may be, it is possible that they are based only on a belief system. I can assure you that, by connecting to the truth through Living Light, those "math problems" blocking your path can be resolved. What that girl managed to do is a perfect representation of what we can do when we believe that nothing is impossible.

To make "the impossible" a reality, it is not enough to affirm that we believe we can do it, given that 90% of our beliefs are unconscious. When we say: "I believe," we are actually saying "I consciously believe," but this is not enough to manifest the physical reality that we would like to co-create. We could spend our days repeating affirmations, but if the circumstances that surround us reactivate painful memories, conscious beliefs are not enough. We end up giving up. We continue to live with our unconscious beliefs without realizing it, and we blame our "failure" on circumstances, instead of blaming our thoughts, feelings and actions; we fall into the energy of blame and self-punishment, faulting our circumstances as the reason for our "problem." Yet it is our belief system that causes this blockage and limits our creative power. We can only transform the system from its origin, from our DNA.

The same memories can bind us to "bad habits," meaning addictions that slowly destroy us. Most habit-breaking experts focus almost exclusively on our conscious thoughts and behavior, which is as difficult as trying to push a very heavy rock up a mountain. To attempt to use sheer free will to end a vice, an addiction, or a bad habit, can lead to a vicious cycle of frustration, wasting too many years of our present incarnation, not to mention risking the possibility of reactivating those habits in the next, or a parallel, life.

For example, in nearly all cases of alcoholism, people are conscious enough to understand and follow the steps to abstain from drinking for a period, but many eventually fail at remaining abstinent. The same thing happens with drugs, cigarettes, sex, food, or any other type of addiction. Working through an addiction can take years, and sometimes it is never overcome; however, sending new information to the cells to drop the habit can unblock the program that generates the vice. By changing the information in the cells, the limiting belief system changes to one of Love and Truth, opening exceptional new abilities in all areas.

Limiting beliefs are responsible for the sabotage of many achievements in life. Sabotage is the number-one creator of all types of excuses that keep us from completing tasks that we deem important. Sustained by the energy of fear, limiting beliefs create excuses that seem as logical and as real as the sun. We believe that someone should have given us something essential for the completion of the task, and they failed do it; or, a situation presents itself at that moment that we judge more important than our original intention; or, suddenly someone very close to us requires our attention. We lay blame everywhere else, claiming that it is they and not us who keeps us from achieving our goals.

All of these things seem real, and they have really happened to us. The important thing is to realize that it is not they who have kept us from completing a task. They are no more than excuses, and these excuses become a vice that becomes a reality, generating new beliefs such as "I have no luck," "I am always sick," or "I could never be in a stable relationship;" in short, we end up living a life that is not the one we want to live.

In reality, it is our limiting beliefs concerning the results we can achieve once we take action, that keep us from carrying them out. When we clear the belief that activates the emotion that limits us and impedes our progress, our rational conscious belief changes automatically. If there are things in our daily life that did not go as we had wanted them to, now we can accept them as such and bring to light all our abilities and talents that allow us to feel our true greatness. Our creative powers no longer have limits, or excuses, since the motivation that activates our belief is transformed into Love.

The cause behind illness and disease in the body is always a limiting belief, and conversely when we transform our emotions into

Love, we access the Truth and then our cells, our DNA, becomes impermeable to disease and illness. When our emotions no longer fit the circumstances that we are living in the present, it is because an old memory is being activated; we are almost never aware that it's a memory causing the emotion, as the feelings are so real that we think the present circumstances are causing them. That is why it is so important to live consciously in the present. Only when we allow the past to emerge do the painful cellular memories reactivate, bringing forth limiting thoughts and feelings.

The reality is that nearly every addiction or destructive habit remains in our DNA, and the beliefs that form and imbed themselves in our cellular memory can be reactivated, causing pain and limitations, keeping us from being able to create our reality from the divine self.

What if we were to stop procrastinating and live the life we've always dreamed of, without limits, recognizing the totality and owning up to the power that exists within us?

Beliefs are so powerful and affect our behavior so profoundly that even what we call a mistake is only a mistake because we believe in "wrong." We can never do anything that goes against our beliefs, since beliefs are the cause behind our actions. It's one thing to want to believe in something but another to truly believe it, and it is impossible to do anything about what we do not believe in. The paradox lies in our unconscious beliefs, those we are not aware of that oppose a conscious belief, generating incoherence that blocks our creative power. That is why we must consciously live the Truth in Loving, live it both consciously and unconsciously, in harmony. That alone results in unequivocal transformation, like the one experienced by the butterfly when it transcends its caterpillar self.

We all can achieve this transformation and take flight on our way to multidimensional evolution, the achievement of mastery, and the perfection of our DNA. No more struggles, no more arguments with ourselves or those around us, trying to prove we are right. The idea is to access that part of the Zero Point Field where initiation of this activation is automatic. We can then heal the cellular memories definitively and permanently and cease to create unconscious blockages. By accepting them and allowing them to be in harmony with All There Is, old beliefs cease to be a problem.

We can cease to exist within the problem, whatever its name may be, whether health, prosperity or relationships. We can live the rest of our lives in a very effective way, addressing our limiting beliefs from the completeness of our DNA.

Beliefs are like radio stations constantly sending out information about themselves, to the point that, after years of listening to the same version, without being able to change the station, we begin to believe and act accordingly. That is why it is necessary to break the cycle, to work from the heart and not from the mind. The mind is the conscious; the heart is the subconscious. There, inside the Eighth Layer of our DNA, lies the major secret. And Love is the vessel that changes this information.

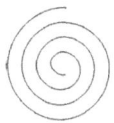

Chapter XVII

The Importance of the Heart

Who looks outside, dreams. Who looks inside, awakens.

Carl Jung

When the heart and mind are in disagreement, we cause an imbalance, or incoherence, in our system. The heart must remain the master and the mind its servant, according to spiritual teacher Osho. When the mind tries to lead, its control takes over what we think, feel, say and do, and this is why it's so important to tune our frequencies into the vibration of Love and allow the heart to command from Truth and Vision. The quantum language experienced in silence is fundamental to the process of balancing and neutralizing the incoherence within us.

There are individuals whose painful memories are deeply rooted; this pain feeds their adrenaline, and such people have difficulty using their imagination and may even lose it altogether. Painful memories, though latent, are ready to emerge to the surface, and this can lead us to unwanted places. That is why it's essential to activate command from the heart, and when we say heart we do not mean the physical muscle but the nuclei of the heart cells, our quantum DNA.

William Thiller is a professor at Stanford University, the author of various books and one of the speakers in the movie What the bleep do we know?! (2004). Thiller, considered by many to be the most prominent quantum physicist of our time, tells us about the importance of intention, which has two faces: our conscious intention and our unconscious intention. We all know conscious intention. Unconscious intention is more elusive; it exists to deal with most of life's issues, drawing from the will of Spirit, of the whole universe, over which the conscious will cannot intervene. The majority of us refer to conscious intention as the most real and essential way to co-create. However, this intention is not the main determinant; whenever conscious intention and unconscious intention conflict, the unconscious eventually prevails.

The universe itself has unconscious intention, which allows for everything to happen, like in the blossoming of a flower that later in the summer becomes a fruit. The flower does not have a conscious intention of becoming a fruit; it is the unconscious intention that exists in the flower, and its connection to the All, that makes it so.

Dr. Bruce Lipton confirms this by declaring that it is almost impossible for us to change our issues using sheer willpower, due to the subconscious mind's being one million times more powerful than conscious will.

By now, I suppose you must be asking yourself: then, what are all of these intentions good for, and all our affirmations and resolutions about what we wish to co-create? If we do not tune them into the Zero Point Field from the energy of Love, then the answer is nothing! It is necessary to transform the pattern of destructive energy anchored in our DNA, which contains the mistaken belief that causes us to be afraid when we should not be; this in turn activates the reactionary system without a logical reason, leading to many types of physical, mental, emotional and spiritual imbalances. To fuse science, spirituality, and art, we have to manifest from the Zero Point Field, where everything is created in the energy of Love.

Therefore, if we wish to free ourselves from physical, mental, emotional, or any other type of health issue, it is essential to add new information — light, color, sound, numbers — to our DNA. We don't do this in a conscious way; we do it by allowing for the synchronicity of creation. Not by giving orders from our existing beliefs, but rather by listening to the most sacred of silences and flowing with the unconscious genius of the cosmos, which is pure Wisdom.

The "Golden Gate" through which the Living Light enters has been predicted by the most lucid scientific minds of our recent times, beginning with Albert Einstein, and has recently become available to the human race. The energy that the limiting programs embed in our DNA can now be healed from the heart. IRB goes beyond that; there is no control. It is about accessing only relevant information.

How great it is to be aware that we still have access to our Original Model, wherein we still experience perfection and total health! In this consciousness, any current imbalance "heals." You, me, all of us, are born into a multidimensional program that authorizes us to make changes the moment we activate it. It is designed to "fix" any imbalance before it becomes a block. Furthermore, if any imbalance presents itself, our program can incorporate a learning from Loving and, in this way, correct it as soon as it appears, without allowing it to become the past and weigh us down as a destructive memory. The simple act of no longer seeing the situation as a problem and changing the perspective from which we observe and live it, is enough for it to no longer exist. It only exists if we give it the power to anchor itself through the energy of fear.

As super beings, we are endowed with all the gifts of Divinity.

However, as long as we believe in falsehoods and live our lives manipulated by the fear that we are limited beings, the files of these gifts become corrupted, causing the program to become slower and slower until eventually it fails. IRB offers us a way to repair the files with the aim of returning to the innate capacity of our being, so the Zero Point Field can allow us access to 100% of the information and to become perfectly balanced, as was designed in the beginning. If we believe that it is possible in a computer, we must begin to see it as something viable in the human model as well.

My spirit was challenged by the message given to us by Kryon, channeled by Marina Mecheva and transcribed at the beginning of this book. Through that challenge, I affirmed my purpose. Since the beginning of time, I have been on a path of healing. That is my main purpose in this incarnation, and I live it every day. I was able to understand that in order to be healthy, it was very important to be in a healing space, asking the right questions with the intention of succeeding. Also, whenever I am anxious or frustrated by distractions, with someone "bothering" or "hurting" me, I can see it as positive. Whether they are just doing their job or not, or becoming an obstacle in my path, all of these elements are part of my path to healing, or better yet, part of my learning and growth.

When I tried to get through the distractions as quickly as possible, I missed some real opportunities for healing, closure and freedom.

As I delved deeper into the concept of healing through the mind, I understood that healing means remaining in perfection within consciousness. If I wish to continue to discover and develop tools of healing to accomplish my purpose, my universe, my world, will continue to have sick people in order for me to accomplish this. Therefore, from that moment on, my purpose became to generate the awareness of flowing from and into the Absolute.

IRB invites us to focus the mind in gratitude when we wake up every morning, aware of the consequences and moving forward in Love to feel the joy of creation at the beginning of each day. It is not so hard to permanently think with a co-creative attitude; it just requires practice. We all have the energy of perfection, we must simply widen the channels that connect us to the dialogue of the most elevated essence of our being to embrace the Living Light that it creates.

It is important to remain present, responding with abundance to anything that the moment offers and being One with whatever we are doing, One with the now, One with the people we serve and who serve us, and One with each thing we co-create.

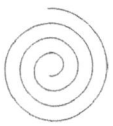

PART THREE

IRB and DNA

Chapter XVIII
The Alchemical Transmutation of Consciousness into Real Life and Purpose

The quantum field responds not to what we want; it responds to who we are being.
Dr. Joe Dispenza

Many protocols have been developed to communicate with DNA and give it the correct instructions for healing humanity. All those attempts have set a wonderful tone for the proper understanding of our DNA: that it is alive, that it conserves our memories, and that it guides our many processes. We have even been able to understand that our DNA communicates in alpha waves, which leads the brain to low and steady cerebral frequencies that facilitate relaxation and the exercise of mental power. Alpha is a sound that the human ear does not catch, but it still allows for harmony and relaxation, thus creating in the brain a state similar to the dreaming state. This is why, whenever we are able to speak in this tone, our DNA obeys our orders. What we haven't previously known is that we are each moment still giving instructions to our DNA based on our current belief system.

In other lifetimes, we have made vows of obedience, chastity, celibacy, poverty and many others, believing at the time that taking verbal religious vows was the best way to reach God. In the same way, when we instruct or command our DNA with words alone, we continue to act from our limiting beliefs.

The radical change that IRB proposes is to not give instructions from our current limited consciousness but to allow our DNA to instruct us, to express itself in its Unlimited divine perfection. The idea is to "listen to our DNA."

Ideally, we are just observers of what is happening. When we attempt to control or explain everything that happens, we are grounding the experience in the mind, which is the home of our limiting beliefs. When we simply accept what is happening, we are freeing our power. Acceptance, then, is the active principle of freedom. Sometimes we want to force events based on what we believe to be right; for example, if we plant an apple seed without knowing that the tree takes three years to come into fruition, we are quickly disappointed. In the first year as the branches begin to grow and thicken, if we are expecting fruit, we may abandon our project to grow apples.

If we decide not to wait around two more years, perhaps someone else will end up reaping the fruit, and continuing to do so for life. This is why it is essential to understand that every moment is a wonderful gift filled with life, even when the manifestation of that life does not look the way we think it should.

To gain a deeper understanding of this, and to generate a broad evolution in our DNA through IRB, we will first do a brief summary of each of the layers that compose our DNA, based on the teachings contained in Kryon XII: The Twelve Layers of our DNA, with additional information provided through the IRB process:

Layer One: *Keter Etz Chayim* – The Tree of Life

כתר עץ חיים

This layer contains all the human genome that, as human incarnates, we possess. Meaning, it contains our genetic heritage: our fathers, grandparents, great-grandparents.... And when we heal their cellular memories, we not only heal our First Layer but that of the next generation, because we prevent the reactivation of the programs contained in that layer, programs acquired during thousands of earlier generations. The First Layer contains chromosomes, the trailers and telomeres that directly affect our physical health and our limitations within the human design.

IRB contains many meditations. Among them is one that we use to activate our light body, permitting us to bring new consciousness to each part of our physical selves to activate the vessel that we use in this incarnation, with the consciousness of a super being. This meditation also leads toward production of a healing hormone from the thymus gland, or high center of the heart, the energetic center that strengthens the highest consciousness of genuine Love.

It is believed that by the age of thirty, in terrestrial linear time, the human cell reaches maturity. By activating our Body of Light, we begin to live in a body that remains in the life force of that cellular maturity at thirty years of age. Kryon tells us that Kether Etz Chayim, "the Tree of Life" in Kabbalistic traditions, contains sephirots, qualities of life associated with each of the principal energetic centers of the human body, widely known as chakras. Traditional science and medicine have always worked on this layer, which was known as the "working" ten percent of our DNA, managing the conventional chemical and physical processes of our body. This is where physical imbalances or illnesses are activated or deactivated on the terrestrial plane.

Layer Two: *Torah E'ser Sphirot* – Programming the Divine Law

תורה עשר ספירות

In this layer we find the Divine Mark that carries our blueprint and allows us to understand what we have come to accomplish in this incarnation, our mission in life. In it we find the programming of spiritual energies, a programming we accomplish before landing in the body we have today. In this layer we also find the original contract that we signed in the bardo, or middle state, or transitional state, as part of our syllabus or lesson plan for this life experience.

This goes hand in hand with Layer Eight. Though they can't exist separately, we explain it in this way because it's simpler; we are accustomed to living every experience in a mixed state, without divisions. It also means, that in the old energy, the duality, it is marked on this plane as the number 2. We will see later on, in the chapter regarding numerology, that in IRB 2 no longer represents duality but rather perfect harmony. When added to Layer Eight, opposites become an indivisible unity, since 2+8 = 10 = 1.

In this layer we find our emotions, which reinforce our thoughts and constitute the fundamental source of our wellbeing or disease, allowing us to neutralize what in Hinduism is called karma, as it allows us to transform learning into pure consciousness.

There's a story of a young girl watching her mother preparing the ham for Christmas, trimming the ends before putting it in the oven. The child asked her mother why she did this, to which her mother replied that it was family tradition. The mother she did not know the reason behind it; all she knew was that her mother had done the same, and the result was the best ham the world.

The girl, restless as are all Indigo Children, called her grandmother on the phone to ask why she cut the tips off the ham, to which she received the same answer: it was a family tradition, and it resulted in the best ham in the world. Her great-grandmother, who was still alive, received the same question, to which the old lady replied: "My dear girl, I always cut off the tips of the ham because the oven in my house is very small, and a whole ham did not fit."

That story reminds us how so many of us repeat behaviors simply because they make up our comfort zone and we believe them to be the right thing to do. That is why Layer Two stores what Eckhart Tolle describes as the "body of pain," which is fed by the history of thoughts and feelings that we remember from our lives, our family, or our race, or our town. It is important to change the concept of karma. Karma is not punishment; it is the effect of a cause that we continue to repeat if we do not incorporate it into this Layer Two of our DNA. The solutions brought by Karma are what moves humanity and what elevates vibration as a whole.

When IRB heals this layer, it heals entire cities and nations; it chooses through consciousness and eliminates karma and punishment and turns them into lessons; it eliminates our addiction to drama in ourselves and our soul families, those who we incarnate with us over and over again until we finally break the Samsara cycle. When this happens, we complete the evolution that allows us to shed our skin.

Layer Two is like our instruction manual; if we listen to it, we can clearly understand the way we must live the present moment to achieve our mission in life. Layer Two continues to present duality in the biological and divine design. It transforms what limits us, what divides us at a level of beliefs and archetypes, it is healing genetic heritage, and when we heal the genetic heritage we are directly affect our Layer One. Though all layers go through our pineal gland, Layer Two governs it.

Layer Three: *Netzach Merkava Eliyahu* - Ascension and Activation

נצח מרכבה אליהו

This layer contains our vessel of ascension, which Drunvalo Melchizedek has named the Merkabah. Layer Three allows us to see ourselves as multidimensional and galactic beings. IRB leads us to transcend the Merkabah to the Merkana, which increases its sacred geometrical complexity from an icosahedron — a polyhedron with two 20 córners, — to the greater light that enables activation of our unlimited vessel of Living Light until it reaches full complexity, the sacred polyhedron of sixty-four tetrahedra. Later we will explain the importance of the tetrahedron, which is the origin of all lifeforms, as illustrated abundantly and masterfully by Nassim Haramein.

Layer Three is itself a catalyst of high frequencies that Kryon invites us to use together with Layer Six (3+6 = 9). The 9 in numerology is the conclusion or ending without things actually coming to an end, but rather evolving. It is vital to transcend the old form, to evolve to a new energy, to a new paradigm of beliefs without limits, to ascend to a new vibration that facilitates the development of the supreme being explained in *The Book of Wisdom: Keys of Enoch*.

Layer Three makes it possible for IRB to be the guidance that opens a state of profound consciousness. This layer activates our dormant potential through the chemistry of the double helix present in Layer One. It is also responsible for keeping us connected to our inner child, hence the importance of re-creating the inner child; not only to connect with him, but to make of him everything we wish him to be.

Do you know what takes place during a magic show? There are two types of adults who attend magic shows: one type that goes with a desire to understand how the tricks work, and when they don't understand, it can ruin their night. They may spend the rest of the evening playing them back in their minds, trying to discover the secret. The second type is children. If they are present at the event, they're simply happy. For them it is not as important to know whether the presentation is magic or illusion; they are just in awe, enjoying everything that happens.

Re-creating the inner child is to never stop being amazed by what life brings us every day without trying to figure out what's behind it, but simply having fun and accepting what is happening. What does it matter if it's a "trick" or not if we allow ourselves to be in awe and enjoy the magic of life? To catalyze the state of joy is one of the greatest gifts of the connection to our inner child, plus a connection to true abundance in life. Layer Three is very present in hypophysis, which produces the magic of visualization and of interdimensional trips. It is the last layer of Group One. There are four groups, each composing of three layers.

Layers Four and Five: *Urim Ve Tumim and Aleph Etz Adonai* - The Cave of Creation

אורים ותומים
אלף עץ אדוני

Kryon explains that Layers Four and Five are inseparable. Of course, as we have already said, in one way or another they are all connected like the rungs of a ladder. If the railing isn't there to hold them together when you climb up or down, you will fall. In IRB, this metaphor means the layers are inseparable because Layer Four, Urim Ve Tumim, is the connection to earth and to our own physical bodies; and Layer Five is our connection to the universe, to our inner Wisdom.

IRB completely connects us to these two opposites and activates them, also activating the center of our heart, allowing us to activate our inner Christ, as we will further study in the summary of Layer Six. Jesus died only to be resurrected; his life was one great metaphor that shows us the exact path to activate the Christ within us, our purest crystalline essence. We must demolish the ego to be resurrected in Presence.

When we activate Layers Four and Five, it is though we climbed into our own spaceship and ascended, meaning we encourage Layer Three to complete its mission, which depends on our Layers Four, Five and Six to become fully resonant. The great evolutionary teacher Peggy Phoenix Dubro, through her knowledge of the Universal Calibration Lattice (UCL®), places special emphasis on the power of "alienation" which she refers to as Bottom Center, Upper Center, and the Heart Center. In practice, this means tuning in and activating Layers Four, Five, and Six, which connect us to what's outside and inside, allowing us to be aware of the power of co-creation in perfect resonance with the Zero Point Field.

Kryon confirms that Levels Four and Five are the essence of expression in this specific life on Earth and divinity on the planet. Which means they constitute absolute union of humanity and God. It is to bind into one sole essence who we truly are. This is why it is so important for connection to Earth to be in complete balance with our connection to superior Wisdom, which empowers us to create by making responsible, wise choices as true Gods. Layers Four and Five, as Kryon explains, represent the name of the crystal in the Akashic registry, are our interdimensional akasha; they tell us who we are and where we have been, not only on Earth, but in other dimensions and galaxies.

Inside the crystal in the cave of creation, we each find our true name. It is our connection to these layers that allows us to know it — to know our true name, not the one we have been given in this incarnation. This is the name by which we are recognized in every corner of the known and unknown universe, which generates within us the power of the One in the All. We can then consider these two inseparable layers the primary attribute of what the tree of life is, found in Layer One, which is the family.

The second group of layers that follows concerns Divinity. Together, they add up to nine. They conclude the mortal reincarnations and rupture the Samsara cycle. When our centers are truly connected, we can emit and live like incarnate angels. We must remember that We Are All one. Nothing is separate. Angels and guides are inside each of us. The only thing we need to understand to experience this truth is to change the vibration of our DNA. When we feel that "God has abandoned us," it is because this change is taking place. We integrate it into our being.

The activation of these two layers grants us power to co-create as humans from divine Spirit. It is the essence of the I Am on Earth; 4 equals light and power; 5 is the same as the essential crystal energy: Love.

It is what activates the Threefold flame in our being.

Layer Six: *Ehyeh Asher Ehyeh* -I Am that I Am

אהיה אשר אהיה

This layer concludes the second group, the Divinity group; it represents in itself the Divinity that Jesus came to teach. Layer Six unites Teacher and God into one being. It is the two-way street of true communication established in meditation and prayer; in meditation we receive information, whereas during prayer we speak.

Layer Six activates communication between Source, or the beings of light, and a human who is becoming a master. When you are able to speak and be heard, you experience true consciousness.

That is the reason Layer Six is the absolute Layer of Consciousness. It helps us understand that we are divine beings and enables us to radiate divinity, sacredness and totality. Peggy Phoenix Dubro, in her previously mentioned UCL® work, uses a beautiful comparison to explain that in the English language, wholeness and holiness sound very similar. When we activate Layer Six of our DNA, we activate our hearts and radiate this sacredness to everything that surrounds us, achieving absolute comprehension of our spiritual being. The heart, not as an organ but as an energetic center, is your Love. It can only be pure Love when we recognize our divine being.

Herein lies the absolute trilogy: Human, God and Teacher. This is what Christ truly came to teach us when he incarnated as Jesus, giving birth to our current era. Therefore, activating and connecting to Layer Six is to activate our inner Christ. Christ means "crystalline," that which does not have a shadow. And when Christ is no longer a person, but an entire race, we evolve, reaching the Christic Race, the Koradi race that can only be activated from Loving. This is the Seventh Race that has already begun to populate the Earth with what we have called Indigo Children, who give life to this potent Indigo Ray. IRB enables us to achieve balance when we synchronize with the Zero Point Field at its maximum expression. Those who wish to find out more about the previous six races that have inhabited the earth can study Blavatsky (188).

In regard to the Seventh Race, in her fourth volume Blavatsky writes:

> The Pauline expression (Hebrews xi. 5) "that he should not see death" — *ut non videret mortem* — has thus an esoteric meaning, but nothing supernatural in it. The mangled interpretation given of some Biblical hints to the effect that Enoch, "whose years will equal those of the world," (of the Solar year, 365 days) will share with Christ and the prophet Elijah the honors and bliss of the last advent and of the destruction of Antichrist–signify esoterically, that some of the great adepts will return in the Seventh Race, when all Error will be made away with, and the advent of TRUTH will be heralded by those *Sishta*, the holy "Sons of Light."
>
> Truly so; the Veda of the earliest Aryans, before it was written down, went forth into every nation of the Atlanto-Lemurians and sowed the first seeds of all the existing old religions. The off-shoots of the never-dying tree of wisdom have scattered their dead leaves even on Judaeo-Christianity. And at the end of the *Kali*, our present age, Vishnu, or the "Everlasting King," will appear as Kalki and re-establish righteousness upon earth. The minds of those who live at that time shall be awakened and become as pellucid as crystal.
>
> It is written: "The men who are thus changed by virtue of that peculiar time (the sixth race) shall be as the seeds of other human beings, and shall give birth to a race who shall follow the laws of the Krita age of purity." Meaning,

it shall be the seventh race, the race of *Buddhas*, the Sons of God, borne of immaculate parents.

To think, feel, speak and act according to the teachings of IRB enables us to become these immaculate parents, these Children of light that create the new crystalline Earth for a new humanity.

As we pointed out during our explanation of Layer Three regarding the metaphor of Jesus's life on Earth, with the activation of Layer Six, IRB enables us to develop the potentials of the inner Christ, the same faculties that the Master Jesus showed during his path on this planet, such as surrendering to God's will. However, we must flow with the unconsciousness of the cosmos that paves the way toward a singular universal purpose. We must know and accept the divine designs; love humanity and all beings; ascend to God; recognize our Original Model; heal sickness and understand that our perfection is a divine reflection; attract substances from the eternal; and forgive our offenses and others', knowing that there is nothing to forgive since everything is part of our learning, facilitating greater evolution and mastery. When we activate this layer, we incorporate in our field the five initiations that Jesus fulfilled during his life: birth, baptism, transfiguration, crucifixion, resurrection and ascension.

There is nothing better than understanding these five initiations, as is explained by the brilliant Spaniard Juan Carlos Garcia in his book Los Cuentos de Hadas en el Cine (Fairytales in the Movies), based on the Disney masterpiece The Lion King.

Birth

"Unless one is born again he cannot see the kingdom of God." (John 3:3).

The Alchemical Transmutation of Consciousness into Real Life and Purpose

At the beginning of the film The Lion King, we see the newborn lion, Simba, heir to his father's kingdom, the source, still unconscious of what he has in the vast empire that he will one day rule. He is mischievous and immature and does not realize the consequences of his actions. He dreams of being a good king, but he forgets the responsibility of his kingdom. It is foretold that he will be a great king and that it was written in the stars the moment he is born. The monkey Rafiki, who is the representation of John the Baptist, and Asita the sage, and so many others in every religious philosophy who have predicted the imminent birth of the divinity incarnate that will redeem humanity, lifts Simba into the air while a ray of light descending from the heavens, bursting through the clouds and surrounding him. All the creatures adore Simba and kneel before him. This epitomizes the moment of worship of the three wise men and shepherds in the life of Christ. Scar, his uncle, is the modern equivalent of Herod. He desires the throne and so conspires to kill the young lion, but without achieving his goal.

The dangers of the physical world: the young lion, not listening to the warnings of his father and other wise beings of his kingdom, enters danger at Scar's suggestion. Scar, who also represents fear, brings Simba into a more dangerous part of his land: the psychic world, or astral plane. Common sense, represented by the toucan Zazu, is ignored, and soon the young prince regrets this.

There everything is dark and menacing. Emotions are heightened and pounce upon the unwary disciple who enters their domain, reawakening inner fears that had lain forgotten at the bottom of the unconscious. The hyenas, representing "negative" emotions sheltered by fear, attack and sarcastically mock Simba. But soon the light from the Presence or Source, in the form of the King Mufasa, intervenes, liberating the disciple from the oppression of this kingdom of illusion and death.

Baptism, Transfiguration, and Crucifixion

After running away to the desert, chased by the hyenas — just as Jesus fled to Egypt to escape Herod — Simba meets a series of characters that could be termed pseudo-instructors, as they possess a very peculiar philosophy of life: Hakuna Matata.

Simba's reunion with Nala, a lioness friend from his childhood, now an adult, symbolizes re-entrance into the spiritual world, lost and forgotten in the solitude of the desert. Nala represents the inner Christ, and this is why Simba joins her, symbolizing the third initiation, the transfiguration. The scene is framed by the beautiful melody Can You Feel the Love Tonight.

Later, Rafiki finds Simba in the field and tells him that his father is not dead, that he still lives inside of him. Rafiki takes him to the river so that Simba can look at his reflection in the water and see within himself. At that moment, the Presence, through his supreme being, is revealed. The heavens open, and we can hear the voice of silence saying: "You have forgotten who you are, and, in forgetting yourself, you have forgotten me. Look inside yourself, you are so much more than what you believe you are. You must take your place in the Circle of life. Remember who you are."

> Luke describes it this way: "And the Holy Spirit descended on him in bodily form, like a dove; and a voice came from heaven: 'You are my beloved Son; with you I am well pleased.'" (English Standard Version, Luke 3:22)

And thus, the human becomes completely in service to the immanent Christ, including the crucifixion and the work of re-conquering the kingdom. In finding our mission, we overcome the fears represented by Scar, the great manipulator, and take back our role in the circle of life, the endless cycle, Eternity.

Resurrection and Ascension

When Nala and the rest ask Rafiki about Simba, he says they will find him back in his kingdom, for he has returned: "Why are you looking among the dead for someone who is alive?" (Luke 24:5)

Simba finds the kingdom in a truly lamentable state. There is no food or divine provisions, and fear has overcome the people. In a fight against sinister forces that hold the kingdom in its grip, Simba and his friends win in the end. Scar, attempting all types of tricks, is devoured by the hyenas, for evil destroys itself. Simba ascends to the throne, and life returns to the kingdom. We now see the landscape adorned in tones of green and blue. All of the creatures greet and salute the new King. The circle of life has been completed.

Layer Six is the conduit, the plumbing, what we know as *Antakarana*, which means: "I am the way, the truth, and life." Beyond being a thread that communicates two separate parts, this is the consciousness of being One, being what the Mayans described as "I am you and you are me," as was explained in Chapter XI. This layer contains the great secret of Moses's code, amply covered in the documentary by James F. Twyman, by reflecting our reality in the other and understanding from a place of Love that we are also the other; Oneness becomes mastery.

Though Layer Six cannot be without the others in its group, Layers Four and Five, they work completely in tune with Layer Three, and both make up the last of their group. In quantum numerology, 6 means communication, balance, and harmony, the characteristics that most resemble the Zero Point Field. This is also why the names of Layers Three and Six are part of mantras that constitute a fundamental part of IRB.

Layer Seven: *Kadumah Elohim* – Divinity Revealed

קדומה אלוהים

This is the first layer of the third group of the Lemurian layers. The Lemuria-Atlanteans were considered to be the First Race; therefore, these layers contain the complete history and accumulated wisdom of this planet. Layers Four and Five connect us to the multi-dimensional Wisdom, permitting Layers Seven, Eight and Nine to act on Earth, guided by Wisdom. Layer Seven is the opposite or, better, is the complement to Layer Six, though it is found in another group.

When we view the illustrations of Ilan Dubro (see http://www.kryonespanol.com/DNA/DNA.html), we see that Layer Six is pink and has a bright golden circle in the center, while Layer Seven is gold with a bright pink circle in the center. This infuses us with the perfected unity of opposites, as between God and Master.

Layer Seven connects us to absolute mastery. Kryon says that it is the Lemurian language given to us by Pleiadians as a divine complement to the normal progression of DNA Earth.

For IRB, this layer is very relevant, as it is through this layer that we connect to the Planetary Unity Grid. When the grid is unified, our DNA becomes an extension of the Earth's DNA. The name of this layer in Lemurian is Hoa-Yawee-Maru, a description of the interdimensional intuitive sense that Lemurians possessed. It is the absolute meaning of Divinity revealed. It is the understanding of true mastery. It was to demonstrate this truth that Jesus incarnated as human, performed great miracles and allowed himself to be crucified — all to tell us that his DNA and ours are the same; the only difference was that he totally believed in his divine nature. So this layer allows us to recognize ourselves as the Masters of Earth. One of the biggest mistakes Christian religions make is to worship Jesus as a God; it is important to follow in the master's footsteps, not to worship him. All the great avatars—or terrestrial incarnations of god—in our history have developed this layer 100% and recognized its divinity, thereby activating their mastery.

Layer Eight: *Rochev Baaravot*-Riders of the Light

רוכב בערבות

Layer Eight, the second of this third group of Lemurian layers, contains our history, the registry of all our past lives, plus parallel and future lives, as well. It also retains all the abilities and talents we have acquired through our many lives and experiences.

The layer that holds the registry of the Masters and permits us to activate self-mastery is, as named by Kryon, the Riders of the Light. In the new energy we are not required to follow anyone. As the great Buddha said, "Be lights unto yourselves. Do not believe something simply because a great guru or master said it, or simply because it is written." Layer Eight is one of the layers given to us by the Pleiadians to complete our divine human design.

The Bible says that when Jesus returns, he will do so on a winged horse; he is the Rider of the Light. This means that the return of Jesus is that of the Christ, our crystalline being, which we attain once Layer Eight of our DNA is fully activated, bringing to the here and now the master attributes that we have gathered in any of our many incarnations. We have gone beyond labeling these incarnations as good or bad; regardless of the role we select to play to further our learning, we develop master attributes that each time bring us closer to our true essence, who we truly are, and all of this is contained within this sacred layer.

The vibration contained in the Lemurian name for this layer is the energy of Wisdom and Responsibility. It's very important when referring to IRB energy to understand that we are 100% free to choose, and we are responsible for the results of our actions. Beyond the karma predicted by the old energy, we must understand that every choice lies dormant in the existing potentials of the quantum field that surrounds us. The relevance of free will is in the Wisdom that assists us from the active mastery, which brings us closer to that reality that we deserve to create as the particles that we are within the great Whole.

IRB transforms carbon into crystal. The body of pain is nested in Layer Eight, along with all the emotions produced in Layer Two. Only an awareness of the power of the present moment can transform the body of pain, as is so clearly explained by Tolle (2006), aided by the master attributes also found in Layer Eight. This is to transform carbon, the essence of all life, into crystal, the manifestation of a more pure reality. One without the other is senseless, and the transformation of one into the other allows us to reclaim our rights to live without limits from our beloved IRB essence, by doing our work from a Loving consciousness, accessing our Akasha, which is found in the perfection of the completeness of our DNA.

Layer Eight allows us to remember that everything is here and that our Wisdom helps us chose the right potential at the right moment. Led by the hand of the master Consciousness, we avoid drowning in suffering in a lesson-based reality where we feel incomplete. We see ourselves only as small, imperfect fractions when actually everything is complete and perfect.

The handling of Layer Eight from Layer Thirteen makes it possible for us to enter the multi-dimension in which the movement of life becomes an internal unfolding, in which everything is simultaneously being lived and recycled, since the universe has the ideas stored in the eternal mind of reflection and revelation. All of the actions in life are stored here to be repeated wisely and to be used by the great masters we are in the superior dimensions, within the infinite worlds of the Lotus consciousness, as Hurtak explains in 1-1-0 of *The Book of Wisdom: The Keys of Enoch*.

Layer Nine: *Shechinah-Esh* – The Flame of Expansion

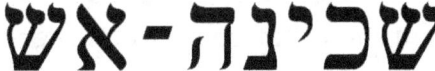

Layer Nine, the third of this third group of Lemurian layers, holds the secret of healing and transmutation; it is the spark that ignites the two previous layers. When we talk about healing in IRB, we are referring to healing the human being, which up until now we have considered "imperfect." The truth is, we must recognize the perfection of everything, ourselves included. We do not heal anything; we understand that there is nothing to heal because we are already perfect. We simply need to choose that reality that is one of the potentials in the field, where illness does not exist, nor lack, nor suffering, since they are part of another reality that we have already lived and, therefore, no longer need to continue to repeat or struggle through. In IRB there is no struggle but only flow, pleasure, love and enlightenment.

Layer Nine is the basic principle of feminine energy from Spirit. The power of creation is implicit in the subtle energy that is Spirit. It contains inside the violet flame, transmutation, transfiguration, what the great St. Germain, avatar of the Golden age, taught through his manifestations of the I Am.

From the Violet Ray comes the Indigo Ray that assists in IRB, offering us the absolute power of transforming what attaches us to the 3D world. In the IRB energy, Layer Nine is able to completely transform fear into Love. We are able to transmute all those feelings in 3D that we call negative, into Living Light, which leads us to being happy in our absolute eternity, wisely choosing the light potentials available in the field for each of us.

When Kryon speaks of the flame of expansion, his meaning is the truth about DNA, which is pure Love. It is the DNA's interdimensional antenna that speaks to Layer One and provides answers from 4D such as pertains to healing. It is the intelligent activation of the human cell. Healing activations takes place through the sound of harmony and silence, balancing the totality of the being and allowing us to understand that the consciousness of Presence is in this layer; that is why it activates 100% of our immune system, to the point that it enables communication with our entire inter-dimensionality.

Layer Ten: *Va-Yik-Ra* --the Call to Divinity

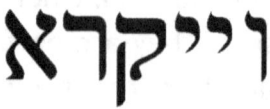

This is the first layer of the group of the Divine Layers, the God Layers. The activation of this group allows us to know our true essence. All religions have taught that we are made in the image and likeness of God. The Divine Layers make it possible for us to activate our Divinity from inside. Layer Ten, called by Kryon "the divine Source of existence," is almost inseparable from Layers Eleven and Twelve, since once it is conjoined with the totality of God, they become the layers of action. Just as we saw that Layers Four and Five are of co-creation, Ten and Eleven set in motion what we co-create with Four and Five, initiating action from profound Wisdom, not from ego. It is important to remember that everything without exception is creation. Chaos is also co-creation, the difference lies in co-creating from the ego or creating from Wisdom, which is given to us by Divinity when we activate our absolute mastery, as we saw in Layers Seven, Eight and Nine.

The attributes of these final three layers are different from those of the previous layers. When Kryon first mentioned them in his channeling from Mount Shasta (2006), he called them invisible layers since they are the divine Source of existence. In conventional numerology, 9 is the highest number; to go higher, we must put an additional number to the right of it. This is why it is in itself an ending. And by ending, as we've already explained, we mean the closing of a cycle in order to begin the evolution of a new one. Va-Yik-Ra represents 10, which in conventional numerology is 1 and, in this case, represents resurrection, as was lived by Jesus after being in "hell," to then take his place on "God's throne."

IRB helps us understand the inner Divinity when we activate this layer. It facilitates enlightenment so that we can remember who we truly are. Going back to previous layers, we could say that Layer Six is the blade that tears open the veil so that Layers Ten, Eleven and Twelve can take it down completely.

Layer Ten activates this consciousness. It has always been there, yet while swimming in it we have not been able to recognize it. We could say it is similar to a fish born in the sea that has never seen the surface, so when asked what the sea is, he doesn't know what to answer; it is so natural to him that he does not know how to differentiate. That is what has happened to us; we have lived eons without knowing it's there. To be able to know Divinity, enjoy it, and make the most of it in its totality, it is important to submerge ourselves completely in this extraordinary layer.

The divine spark that we are permanently connected to, lights the flame called Va-Yik-Ra, which is willingness to work overtime so that our beloved supreme essence, the highest part of ourselves, can find a way to connect us to the Truth. This is a Truth that will never abandon us again, not ever, not even for a minute. On the contrary, it begins to lay a foundation more beautiful than anything we have ever imagined. These layers can only be activated in their totality with the intention that comes from Love.

Layer Eleven: *Chochma Micha Halelu* - Wisdom of the Divine Feminine

חוכמה מיכה הללו

Layer Eleven is the second of the group of divine layers, representative of the creative self. This is the mother who gives life to creation, the feminine energy whom religion has tried to suppress for eons. It is the womb, absolute creation. It is wisdom from creativity, from femininity. It is not about the goddess energy, since it goes beyond feminine energy; it is the Wisdom of the Divine feminine. It is transcendence. It is the energy of pure Compassion. It is the third energy that is created between the feminine and masculine to achieve balance, the purest balance in duality.

The era of Pisces was about patriarchal heritage, worship of the masculine. Woman, in her urge to be "equal," has worked tirelessly to become just as masculine as men. She forgot her essence, her inner truth, her intuition, her inspiration, her creativity; she engaged in a relentless race to compete with masculinity and thus separated herself from her essence, injecting even more masculinity into society, family and the nucleus, further anchoring the patriarchal. On this path, she created all manner of disease in her body, because she forgot about the power that creates illness. This brought on uterine, ovarian and breast cancer, due to the rejections of the body, of her essence. The activation of Layer Eleven is the return of true balance to Earth.

IRB is born in this era of light and rebirth to connect people, whether men or women, with their true essence, to heal the history of nations and its people, to reflect the DNA of humanity, to break free of old patterns, and to let go of old paradigms. Layer Eleven is the fundamental tool that allows us to introduce the new paradigm. IRB vibrates with the number 11, the angelic number, and it takes us to 13, the number of the purest Love; 11 means enlightenment.

Layer Twelve: *El Shadai* - God

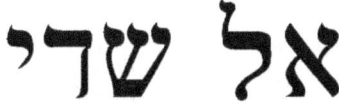

This is the third God Layer of the Divine Group and very important to consider as part of Layers Ten and Eleven, since the three represent action and, considered together, are absolutely different from the previous nine. Kryon describes the Twelfth Layer as the simplest layer because it is the most divine. It is the inner God, the last of the final group formed by God and the one with the highest vibration. Layer Twelve does nothing on its own but only offers peace and refuge; it makes us feel at home.

To be able to create in the present the same way that our Divine Wisdom does, it is necessary to get rid of the old patterns contained in Layer Eight; through the power of Layer Eleven, we activate the master attributes contained there and obtain the peace that cleanses and clears everything we see. When we are able to change the future, we can create the present we want. This is achieved only in one state of consciousness, that which leads us to believe that we are capable of creating, and if we are capable of creating, we are also capable of transcending. That is why it is so important to act from divine Consciousness.

Layers Three, Six, Nine and Twelve are the compendium of Everything that is, the final layer of each group; when activated simultaneously they break barriers and, going through our own consciousness, lead us to understand ourselves as multidimensional beings. Layer Twelve, the Shadai, is the pure layer of oneness. It does not activate on its own but only gives us the awareness to do it ourselves. It is the layer that opens a spectrum of memories that we can use to once again touch our origin. It reminds us that we came from God, that everything is God, and that we are part of Everything. It opens the door to the understanding of our new paradigm.

Layer Thirteen: *Shem Ha-Mephorash* - The Quantum Orchestrator

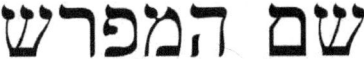

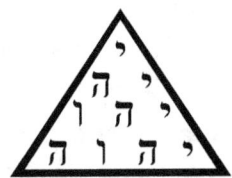

According to Hurtak (2005), Shem Ha-Mephorash is the Tetragrammaton that is never spoken of but remains sacred. It is the ineffable divine name. This name blesses and governs all human interactions with the inner mysteries of life, protecting the future evolution of our DNA. This future is here and now. The moment of evolution is coming through IRB. This name is Name Number 58 of God, and this number also adds to thirteen.

Layer Thirteen is the connector that joins all the parts. This layer makes it possible for all of the ingredients to become a recipe. The alchemist takes the unique individual flavor of each ingredient and mixes all of them together, creating the most exquisite dish. They are no longer separate ingredients but part of the All. When combined, they create something unique. Layer Thirteen is the director of the orchestra, the quantum orchestrator. We know what the twelve basic instruments of the orchestra are and what they sound like, but without a director, no matter how tuned they are, they just play separately, each with its own tone and melody. Layer Thirteen leads them into a beautiful symphony never before heard by the universe. In this way, it guides us toward achieving transcendence and materializing the potential of all the other layers. Layer Thirteen leads us to a new reality, the manifestation of the consciousness of Layer Twelve combined with the virtues of the rest.

There are currently processes that connect us to Layer Twelve, tuning us into the existing information of the fourth dimension. Starting from the fifth dimension, we can go through the portal into everything that is. Activating Layer Thirteen connects us with the All, beyond mastery and Divinity, accessing multidimensionality. It's the consciousness of "Being" rather than that of "being somewhere," transcending even the present. The present gives us the consciousness of spiral time, as the Mayans taught us, and when we go into said heightened state of consciousness, we transcend this limited present that in one way or another keeps us anchored in time.

If we do away with time, what is left is the being, the essence. We can go even beyond the concept of Love. There is nothing more to heal. There are no opposites and no duality; there is only complete Oneness. Everything is. There is no choice to make. Everything is beyond Love; it is essence; it is infinity. All the way up to Layer Twelve, we still find duality, and when we tune into Wisdom, our choices are made from Divinity. However, when we activate Layer Thirteen, there is no longer any duality; there is only the essence of being. It is the truth and the Living Light that transmutes our perception, generating the chaos that gives birth to a new perspective from totality.

Perception occurs at a much more fundamental level that transcends matter: the world of quantum particles. We do not see reality per se, only it's quantum information and, from there, we put together an image of the dimension we find ourselves in. Then we take a step back to contemplate the All from our true essence. It is the Point Zero in the full magnitude of its purest essence. To perceive the world is to tune into the Point Zero Field from Layer Thirteen of our DNA.

The Alchemical Transmutation of Consciousness into Real Life and Purpose

It is the sacred sound generated inside each being responding to the call to restructure and complete the DNA, giving us the ability to identify our own sound, the inner sound that coordinates our DNA, remembering the unique and original characteristics that we have as part of the infinite orchestra of the universe. It is the sound that transforms us. It is accessing the morphogenetic field where the hologram of who we really are, manifests in the dimension we find ourselves in.

It is to activate cell by cell without loss of energy, to distribute the frequencies of the Zero Point Field mirrored in own body, creating a physical "internet" inside of it that links to the outside. It is to communicate through the quantum inner process IRB creates in our being, allowing us to reach coherence as it penetrates the nuclear energy found in the nucleus, in the purest DNA, which produces the collective cooperation and explains internally the unification of thought and consciousness.

When we tune into our divine process through IRB, the coherence becomes contagious, going from the individual to the groups and exceeding the capacity of any known connection to this point in our dimension, earth. It accesses a harmony that resonates with each individual and entire communities, with the highest and most elevated supreme essence of our being. This is regardless of location because, just like the lotus flower, it exists in its purest state despite its surrounding. In other words, lying in a predetermined individual state, it remains in a quantum state, a condition before all other possible states. It can choose the potential quantum state and permanently modify it from the totality to which it belongs. It can then create a coherent energy in conjunction with other individuals, unifying mind and matter through Spirit, codifying the existing information in the Zero Point and transmitting it everywhere at once.

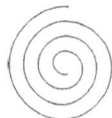

For more information and free gifts go to IRB —
Transforming Fear Into Love
bit.ly/XimenaDuqueValencia_IRB

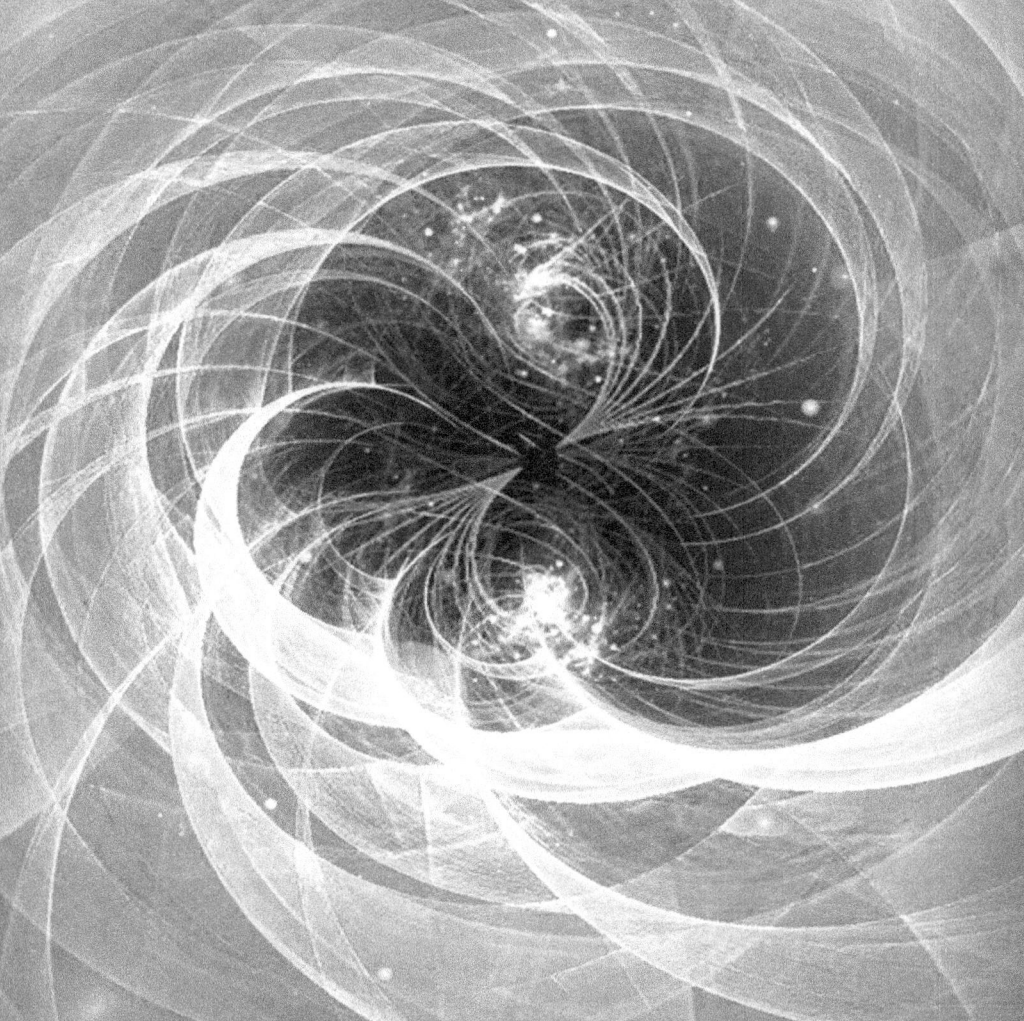

Chapter XIX
The Zero Point Field

If a person practices three qualities, he or she can become One with All. Others will experience Divinity through you. The three qualities begin with P and are: Purity, Patience, and Perseverance. Whoever possesses these three qualities will be free of fear wherever they are.

Sai Baba

The Zero Point Field, which from now on we will refer to as ZPF, is formed by an infinite number of waves of information that are always available to us. This Field is a great storage locker containing realities and sacred memories. IRB, by setting into action Layer Thirteen of the DNA, prepares us to gain unlimited access to these frequencies, based on a mathematical formula set forth in the IRB workshop that guides this project. In a channeling with Kryon experienced through Marina Mecheva at the beginning of 2013, Kryon described it as "a project so powerful, so life-changing, so capable of transforming realities [...]."

When we allow ourselves to interact consciously with the ZPF, we activate intuition and creativity at 100% percent, gaining a clearer understanding of what until now were thought of as "miracles." This suggests, as Hurtak says in The Book of Knowledge: The Keys of Enoch, that when we take our super-being-like capabilities toward knowledge and communication at a level much deeper and extensive than we can understand right now, our sense of separation vanishes. When we access ZPF, we lose sight of where we end and the rest of the world begins; Consciousness exists between the field and ourselves.

There is no longer an "out there." Everything is interconnected, not only at the level of knowing but at the level of experiencing, of having manifest awareness of the imminent event. This is such a vast concept that is hard to understand from a book. It is necessary to begin to live it to know its completeness. We must begin to exchange such energy, to structure Layer Thirteen so that we can open all types of possibilities in relation to the universe from the ZPF and Layer Thirteen of the DNA. If we allow ourselves to continue asking how or why, we will continue to delay our evolution, as scientists have done for decades. If we continue to ignore the effect of IRB within the ZPF, we eliminate the possibility of an interconnection, overshadowing what we call miracles, from a limited explanation that removes God from us.

Let us remember, as is explained in Chapter VII, that any great change in the world of thought comes from many minds beginning to raise questions at the same time. In the same way, reality emerges from the ZPF with the participation of a living consciousness; nothing exists independent of our perception of it. Consciousness itself creates order, meaning it creates the world and its interrelationships. If reality is the result of the interaction of consciousness with its surroundings, consciousness lives in a world of unlimited possibilities.

When our ZPF clears the limiting old patterns and everything that holds it back, it creates a great impact on the consciousness. It allows willing access from a place of Love — not fear, greed or competition — to all the infinite and unlimited potentials offered by the ZPF.

The Zero Point Field

Quantum physics (as elaborated by Louis de Broglie, a French physicist awarded in the 1929 Nobel Prize in Physics for his discovery of the wave nature of the electron, known as the De Broglie Hypothesis) concludes that the "individual consciousness has its own 'particular' separation, but it is also able to behave as a 'wave' through which it can flow through any barrier or distance, to exchange information and interact with the physical world."

IRB invites us to surrender our individual identity for a major, vastly more complex entity in order for the most elevated essence of our being to develop greater coherence. If we attempt to do this individually, we will succeed, but if we do it with someone with whom we share profound feelings, this has a much more powerful effect. So, then, if the effects for a couple are so potent, what would happen if we did the same thing as a mass? The effect depends on the resonance of consciousness of those who participate, and the more intense effects are produced among people who share identities — and I need to explain that this has nothing to do with consciousness. It is our essence that has the capacity to communicate with the physical yet sub-tangible world, that quantum world that contains all possibilities and is capable of generating something so tangible in the manifest world.

The unconscious mind is the world before thoughts and conscious intention. The ZPF is the inconsistent matter that exists in the probabilistic state of all possibilities. Synchronicity, or the resonance between these two states, is the maximum power of co-creation, which we achieve by going deeper into the quantum world, where there is no difference between the mental and physical states. This difference is what is considered as realistic and separatist thinking. To operate in this conscious state of unity is simply to make sense of the stream of information, where two worlds don't exist but only one: the ZPF and the ability of mass to organize itself coherently.

IRB tunes us into the awareness of being a rippling waterfall of individual quantum coherence that allows us to act as a single unit, reflected in the ZPF, extending to the world from the unity of coherent thought.

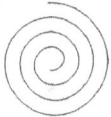

Chapter XX

The Vessels of Transformation

All shallow roots must be uprooted because they are not deep enough to hold you!

Helen Schucman

1. Pineal Gland

When we transcend our physical senses, seeing beyond the 3D world, perhaps even seeing the future, listening to octaves unreachable to the naked ear, communicating without need of 3D language, using telepathy, moving objects with telekinesis, and so on — all of this comes from what is described as the third eye, also commonly referred to as the sixth sense. In reality, it goes beyond six: once again the number 13 is relevant to our history, since the activation of this gland leads us to accessing thirteen senses, many of them unknown.

The pineal gland has been a great mystery for centuries. It is located approximately in the middle of the head and, as says David Wilcock, one of the main developers of this idea in our current era, is the access point of our astral body and our physical body.

It is a reddish-violet color and is the point where all the information of the universe enters, despite being the size of a pea (when it should really be the size of a golf ball) and shaped like a pine cone or an ear, which forms are part of the iconography of many philosophies and religions of the world.

According to surgeons, the gland has an opening with a lens to distinguish light; it is hollow and has receptors to distinguish colors; it has 90° vision. The only direction it cannot see is down.

Defenders of the pineal gland such as David Wilcock confirm that within this gland we find water molecules capable of very sharp reception of universal vibrational frequencies, and of decoding the geometry and mysteries of how reality was created. This understanding is in all of us, recorded in our DNA, but in the "fall" (when we changed from harmonious consciousness to a non-harmonious one), we forgot it, and without these memories, we begin to breathe differently. That is why the main objective of IRB is to activate your balance, where 100% of the information is recorded.

Breathing is essential to living, and to remembering that we are Consciousness, as well. Pranic energy, or the energy of life, originally circulated through the center of the pineal gland, but as this powerful gland calcifies due to fluoride and other manipulations of our water and food supply, it stops using its prana, the vital energy of the universe. Prana has effectively ceased to come through the pineal gland and circulate through our system. It is said that this is the main reason why, when we started breathing through our nose and mouth, we began perceiving reality as good or bad; meaning, duality was created as a reality, though it is only an illusion created by incorrect inhalation of prana. Let us consider that by activating the totality of our DNA we can remember once again how to breathe through our pineal gland, partaking of the prana of the universe.

Hinduism explains that not having our vital energy go through our third eye causes us to no longer see things as they really are, and we are presented with an alternate reality, or perhaps a different interpretation, which we know as polarized consciousness, or the consciousness of right and wrong. The results of this make us mistakenly believe that we are inside looking out, separated from everything outside of us.

We can restore the prana, or vital energy, through the pineal gland through an ancient Atlantean initiation inherited by the Egyptians, who were experts in this modality. This technique, besides activating the pineal gland, activates the body of light all human being bring with them at the moment of birth. This practice has been shared in IRB seminars that began officially in 2014 in Colombia. You can access these events through the following link: bit.ly/XimenaDuqueValencia_IRB

The body of light is the medium through which the highest essence of our being tunes into the totality of who and what we are, carrying the information of our Akashic records, in which we share each manifestation of life that we experience. The memory of who we are before and after every life experience, is related to the pineal gland.

Initiation in the ancient Atlantean mysteries activates the pineal gland and the body of light, and we acquire a consciousness of immortality that enables us to remember our past life experiences, and we can, with wisdom and compassion, incorporate into our present experience everything we have learned. This is true immortality, when we are able to return home using the body of light connected to the pineal gland.

IRB allows us to evolve at a frequency where all of our gifts, including clairvoyance, become a part of our day-to-day experience. For some, this is a gift that comes naturally, such as for the Indigo Children. For others, it is a longer journey. In the old energy, near-death experiences were necessary, or hits to the head or to the coccyx, or the use of entheogens (vegetable substances that when digested set off a divine experience — thus the meaning behind "God is within us," provoking trance states or shamanic possession in those who consume it, when they find themselves inspired and possessed by the energy that has entered their body).

These states are associated with prophetic trance, erotic passion, artistic creation and religious rituals in which mystical states are experienced through consuming substances trans-substantial with deity. There is also a connection with the opening of Kundalini energies that elevate the potential of our being. Now, with IRB, it is done naturally. With the simple connection to the field, our potential reveals itself within the supreme perfection of Adam Kadmon, the Primitive Man, the Divine Man.

To delve deeper into the history of the pineal gland and its sacredness throughout history and religions that include Hinduism, the Egyptians, the Vatican, and the Masons, it is best to read works by historian David Wilcock, an expert on this potent organ.

Speaking in medical terms, the pineal gland has four main functions: it induces sleep; it converts signals from the nervous system into endocrine signals; it regulates endocrine functions and secretes melatonin, a hormone which helps regulate the process of puberty; and it protects the body cells from harm caused by free radicals.

By putting fluoride in our water and other vital elements of daily consumption, we inhibit these functions while increasing the use of pharmaceuticals that activate the production of melatonin artificially, making our organism function but not develop, instead needing more of these pharmaceuticals, making us codependent and even robots of manipulation.

This small gland has awakened the attention of great thinkers and the enlightened since time immemorial. So then, why has the manipulative Elite tried to promote the inhibition of this gland during history? Why does this Elite possess vital information only to keep it hidden? Why can't most people simply use their pineal gland to "see?"

Before 1990, no significant research had been conducted on the pineal gland. That year Dr. Jennifer Luke, from the University of Surrey in England, arrived to the meticulous conclusion that the pineal gland is the primary target of fluoride accumulation in the body. The soft tissue in an adult gland contains more fluoride than any other tissue in the body, close to 300 ppm, with the ability to deactivate enzymes. The gland also contains hard tissue (hyroxyapatite crystals), a tissue that accumulates even more fluoride, almost 21,000 ppm more than it should. After this finding, Dr. Luke dedicated herself to experimenting with animals to determine how the utilization of fluoride can affect the functioning of the pineal gland, mainly the gland's regulation of melatonin. Results showed that animals treated with fluoride showed reduced levels of melatonin in their urine. This, along with early onset of puberty in the fluoride-treated female animals. Luke summarized her human and animal findings as follows:

> In conclusion, the human pineal gland contains the highest concentration of fluoride in the body. Fluoride is associated with depressed pineal melatonin synthesis by prepubertal gerbils and an accelerated onset of sexual maturation in the female gerbil. The results strengthen the hypothesis that the pineal has a role in the timing of the onset of puberty. Whether or not fluoride interferes with pineal function in humans requires further investigation.

Each day, world corporations are increasingly manipulated to adopt the use of fluoride in public drinking water and in first-aid items. This is why it is necessary to live with organic consciousness, to facilitate the direct connection with our supreme essence through the Totality of what we are, and stop making room for these exterior factors whose purpose is to keep us stupid.

When we know the truth, we can live in peace and stop being manipulated and living with half-truths. The decalcification and activation of the pineal gland reminds us of the legend of the Phoenix bird, a mythical creature told about in many cultures, from Egyptian to Catholic in different versions. This legend is representative of the activation of our pineal gland.

The sun cannot be seen when it is nighttime, and darkness blossoms. Metaphorically, the sun dies at night and is reborn in the morning, like the Phoenix, as represented by the pineal gland. According to an Egyptian legend, a sacred temple in the city of Heliopolis was built in honor of the Phoenix so that she would return every 500 years, to die then come back from its own ashes. Now that the 26,000 years of darkness are over, the night can end and the galactic dawn can bring the sun back.

THIS IS THE TIME for the pineal gland to return to its origin, after having been burned and calcified, and for it to return strong, as a new Phoenix, activating all the knowledge it obtained from its origins, so that a new cycle of inspiration can begin.

The first Christians, influenced by Hellenic cults, believed that in Eden under the tree of forbidden fruit, a rosebush blossomed. There, along with the first rose, a bird was born with spectacular feathers and an incomparable song; this was the only being that did not want to taste the fruit of the forbidden tree. When Adam and Eve were exiled from paradise, a spark from the sword of a cherub fell on the nest and the bird burned instantly. But from its ashes, a new bird emerged, one with incomparable plumage, scarlet feathers and a golden body. Immortality was the reward for its devotion to the divine precept, along with other gifts such as knowledge, healing power in its tears, and amazing strength.

IRB allows us to activate our wings with colors, sounds, rebirth and immortality, through the pineal gland.

The Vessels of Transformation

THIS IS THE TIME to start over, despite having lived in difficult situations; this is the time to change the way we see things, to be reborn physically and spiritually, from the power of fire, purification and immortality.

The pineal gland is also associated with the legend of Onphalos, a word in Greek mythology referring to the navel, considered in ancient times the symbol for the center. From this center, the world is created. The pineal gland is located in the center of the brain and is responsible for the creation of our own world. Whatever we believe we can create, it is possible to do so through this "cranial navel." In the legend, Onphalos could be found in the Delphi Museum. It was a pineapple or egg-shaped stone found with the engravings of the silhouette of the tree of life, plus interwoven infinity symbols which we will talk about later in the book. The legend says that Zeus sent two eagles to opposite sides of the universe. The eagles found themselves in Delphi, where Onphalos marks the spot, becoming the symbol for the center, the place where the creation of the world begins.

In the Bible we find a phrase, "The eye is the lamp of the body. If your eyes are healthy, your whole body will be full of light." (Matthew 6:22) This refers to the pineal gland, the third eye, the eye that sees everything, that can transcend earthly senses and that, when it is activated, fills our vessel of communication with light, with the most supreme essence of our being, permitting us to go into the ZPF of original creation.

According to Sufi medicine, the pineal gland needs natural light for it to work adequately, so the connection with nature and with the sun will greatly help its activation as it fully accesses IRB, where we find complete joy, allowing us to be balanced.

The Pineal gland has all the properties of a quartz crystal; therefore, it has the ability to produce the necessary spark to ignite the flame of illumination. There is a phenomenon called piezoelectricity, present in certain crystals; when subjected to pressure or tension, they become polarized, the same phenomenon that causes a lighter to ignite a spark. The piezoelectric effect is normally reversible; when you stop subjecting the crystals to an external voltage or electric field, they regain their shape. The pineal gland has the same characteristics as quartz and tourmaline, which is why, when it makes contact with certain fluids, vibrations are transmitted and ultrasound is produced. This makes it so we generate our own sound, which elevates high vibrations to the highest frequencies ever imagined, to connect us to the most sacred essence of our being.

When we produce our own sound, we build the high voltage necessary for the spark, not unlike the click produced by a lighter. When we ignite the spark in our pineal gland, we tune into the frequency that produces a resonance at maximum oscillation, and a radiant inner flame is produced that fills our entire vessel so that we experience the totality of our cells, and the totality of our DNA. IRB activates the sound from a powerful mantra centralized in one of its nuclear commands, which will be explained later.

The Indigo Ray possesses a frequency that permits the activation of the DMT crystals, calcium and other waters found in the pineal gland. When this gland comes into contact with the Indigo Ray, the molecules of the crystal are freed and emit light photons, creating millions of colors that we have yet to see in 3D. We experience the new realities and the past, present, and future contained in the Akashic record of all the civilizations of light that have ever lived on Earth, and incorporate this superior Wisdom within ourselves, finally living without the manipulation of linear time, in the eternal present.

Every physical body or system operates at characteristic frequencies. When a system tunes into the specific frequency, its vibration is at its fullest potential. For example, when we tune into a radio station, we put to work an inner circuit of a determined frequency that resonates with the station, amplifying it and permitting it to be heard. When a physical system is submitted to that stimulus of energy, a determined frequency is created with maximum possible absorption; this can lead to the rupture of a point within it, as has happened when a soprano shatters a glass by reaching a particularly high note, which is none other than the glass's own resonating frequency.

Activating our own frequency keeps us from coinciding with other frequencies that could affect us, tuning instead into those that create a reality from Living Light. It is not about protecting ourselves from anything, but rather simply not being exposed to the frequencies that may disserve us. Initiation into IRB permits us to the individual frequency that unifies us with oneness.

In the Key 1-1-0 of the Book of Knowledge of All Kingdoms, Hurtak writes that when we interconnect to the Egyptian language with Hebrew, Sanskrit, Tibetan, and Chinese, we are able to open our minds to the inner light, activating pictographic communication within the brain. The information that IRB brings in its music is a template that unifies these five languages and turns them into mantric music, in sacred energy sounds that activate Living Light ways of thinking that connect to the superior Wisdom unifying human and God through a unique, illuminated cosmic vibration.

Once the pineal gland is activated with this music (sacred sounds) which makes this key possible, it becomes permanent once we facilitate the vertical and horizontal patterns through the divine vector created by the focused light force that forms the necessary links to connect to the inner dimensions of sensorial perception with the superior dimensions that offer infinite pleasure. What IRB achieves in this step is to open us to the Presence of the evolutionary model that offers us the divine power of Living Light.

The name of Layer Thirteen is also of Hebrew nature, as is the Twelfth before it, so as to achieve the final balance necessary to connect our current hologram to the Original Model of Adam Kadmon, who from now on we will refer to as OMAK, with models of Redeeming Creation permitting us to cross the Alpha and the Omega into a new creation.

2. The Tetrahedron as the Basis of Sacred Geometry

The tetrahedron is one of the forms making up sacred geometry. It is also one of the Platonic solids. Through sacred geometry we can experience a simpler understanding of the profound connection that exists in all creation, as it is a symbolic language of the universe that permits us to understand what we intuitively know.

The whole of the universe comes from one Source, or Universal Intelligence, regardless of whether the label given is God, Mother Nature, Great Spirit, Cosmos, Source, Spirit, or just Being. Sacred geometry shows us, with concepts that we can understand with our rational mind, how everything that exists is created by the same basic principles, from an atom to a galaxy. Everything in nature, in the universe, follows the same geometric patterns.

In each manifestation of life, whether mineral, vegetable, or animal, we see triangles, circles, hexagons, ellipses, and spirals. Millions of years on earth elapsed before we could discover the similarities among creatures on earth and group them into fundamental patterns.

The Vessels of Transformation

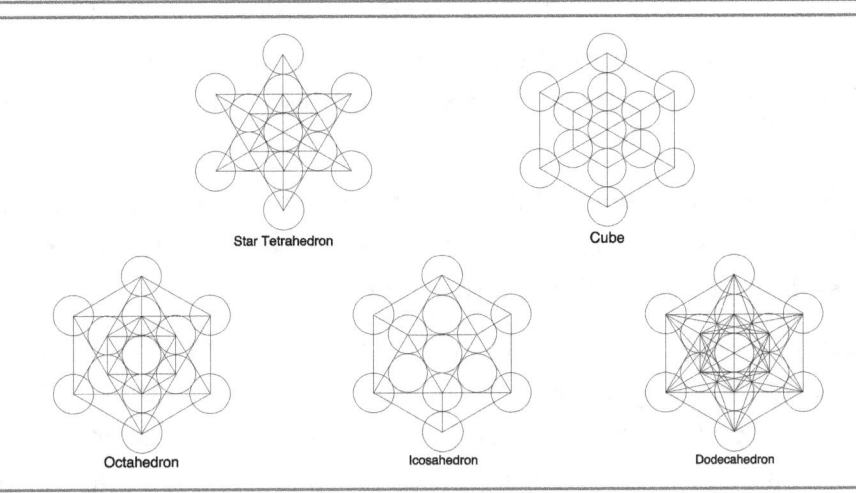

Star Tetrahedron • Cube • Octahedron • Icosahedron • Dodecahedron

There are seven principal shapes in sacred geometry: the five platonic solids, the circle and the spiral.

The five platonic solids are: the tetrahedron, the cube, the octahedron, the dodecahedron and the icosahedron, perfectly symmetrical shapes that all contain the same number sides and angles, and the same measurements. Also the five fit into the universal matrix that is the sphere.

The tetrahedron, which is a triangle at its base, represents fire consciousness. It has six edges, four triangular faces and four vertices. It is the symbol of Wisdom due to its representing the sacred fire, the first element. It contains all potential sexual energy, conceived as divine energy rather than the pleasure of the senses.

The cube, with twelve edges, six square faces and eight vertices, represents the secret of the natural world. It is Earth Consciousness, the experience of that which has been born from nature.

The octahedron has twelve edges, eight triangular faces and six vertices, and looks like two inverted pyramids joined at the base. It is the air element. It symbolizes the perfection of matter through Spirit.

The dodecahedron has thirty edges, twelve pentagonal faces and twenty vertices, and represents the fifth element (ether, prana, chi, or ki). It is considered the feminine power of creation and the mother form.

The icosahedron, with thirty edges, twenty triangle faces and twelve vertices, is water consciousness. It represents the seed of life, the form of the universal masculine.

Creation engages in play by transforming from one shape to another, generating a rhythm and sacred dance in the exchange of the masculine icosahedron and the feminine dodecahedron, while it passes and re-creates the other platonic solids, generating planetary grids and morphogenetic fields that are the sustaining matrixes of all existing forms. The grid stores the information that comes through a member of a species and makes it available to other members of that species, as explained in the chapter on the theory of the hundredth monkey. This concept is not a new one, as Plato theorized about it, as did the Mayans, the Egyptians, the Hopi Indians and many others. These grids group together and relate through the geometric structures of the platonic solids, which is the same formula from which we all derived, proving that we are all truly One.

Earth is surrounded by an electromagnetic grid made up of a matrix of sacred geometry. Plato said that the basic structure of Earth can be found in the process of evolution to an icosahedric grid (of twenty triangles). These matrixes are grids that cover our entire planet, our body, our places, our cells, and atoms, modulating the pattern that holds and creates each form. They are of Crystalline origin, imperceptible to human vision, and move at the speed of light, sending information in its own language, facilitating our development through a teaching method that has no need for books or intellect. Said language is made up of 144,000 seals of crystalline energy—the way that light is decoded—and creates a Christic consciousness on Earth.

Beyond the series of platonic solids, there exists another geometric form that is generated from the ancient icosa-dodecahedron crystal (the union of feminine-masculine). This is the grid that evolves the planet, creating a resonance of superior frequencies that elevate the state of consciousness toward a new existential scale. This resonance comes through the Indigo Ray, which offers from the tetrahedron base a new grid, a Merkabah evolved to an endless number of polyhedral forms.

The sphere is a pattern of unity into which all forms and grids unify; though each has its own characteristics and interconnections. Each conserves the exclusive properties of its individuality and the solid it represents. They all unify in the Source from which they all come.

The planet goes through well-known dramatic changes in climate over time; even the migration patterns of birds are changing; likewise, the electromagnetic Field of Earth goes through changes. The new grid of consciousness increments its frequency as the magnetic grid weakens. The old grid disappears as the new pure crystal matrix is forming. We are all part of this new Christic formation.

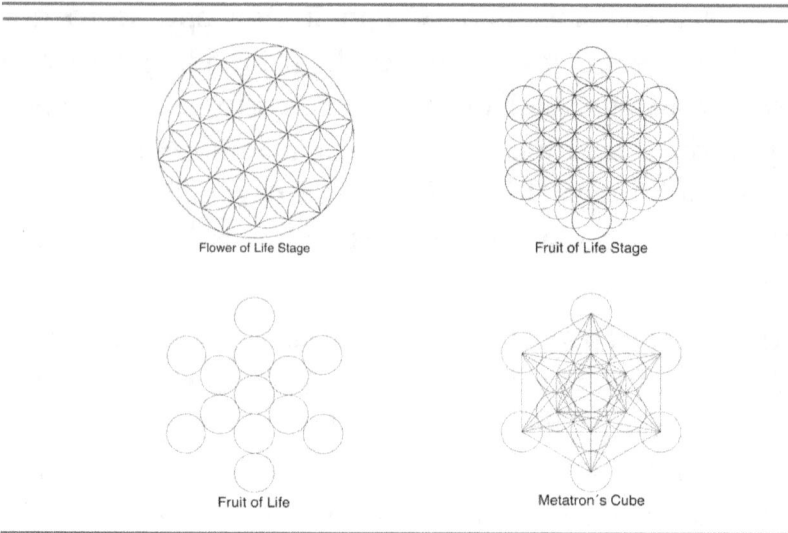

Flower of Life Stage Fruit of Life Stage

Fruit of Life Metatron's Cube

The sacred geometry of the crystalline planetary grid contains the patterns of the Flower of Life, which is the matrix of creation. The Flower of Life is the holographic code of all design in creation and every manifestation in the universe. This code is what creates, expands and develops all life manifestations. What exists, what is, is born from this divine matrix. This hologram represents the spherical geometric sequence, a unity conformed of infinite, evenly-spaced, overlapping circles that form the shape of the Flower of Life.

The Flower of Life is made up of infinite codes of color, sound, and geometric shape through which each atom of life is designed and expressed. Each cell of our being contains information of perfection, of universal memory, and of the harmony and abundance contained within the OMAK.

By activating the OMAK in our current hologram, we restore any part that is in disharmony, establishing balance and restoring youth and perfect health to the totality of our being.

IRB permits the conscious design of the hologram as a symbol of perfection in these moments, on the indigo planet. The human being is the Flower of Life itself.

When we are capable of understanding, from the micro-cosmos to the macro-cosmos, holograms, fractals and spirals, we create the miracle of One.

Haramein proposes a fractal structure that explains the source of creation of all things we know, including humans, animals, planets and the universe itself, through the implicit uniqueness of the tetrahedron. All these theories are currently being studied by NASA scientists to investigate what Nassim proposed.

Additionally, Haramein's work supports the theory that everything in the universe is connected, from the biggest to the smallest scale, through the unified compression of gravity. He proves that it is space that defines matter, not matter that defines space. Haramein says:

> Remember that matter is made up of 99.9 percent space. Quantum field theory states that the structure of space-time itself, at the extremely small level, vibrates with tremendous intensity. If we were to extract even a small percentage of all the energy held within the vibrations present in the space inside your little finger, it would represent enough energy to supply the world's needs for hundreds of years. This new discovery has the potential to open up, access and harness that energy like never before, which would revolutionize life as we know it today.

IRB bases its purpose on this creative tetrahedral basis that is born from the most sacred fundamental structure, to reach more complex and unlimited structures that permit us to travel through the multi-dimension without limits, in complete Oneness.

On the other hand, since before we can even remember, mandalas or psychograms have been used as tools for meditation, concentration and even healing. The meditator's thoughts are guided to find the way to his or her inner self through iconographic images, and thus find self-realization. In other cultures, geometric shapes are used to create magnetic and energetic fields that are attributed with protective powers.

IRB has designed a strategy through the mandala of sacred geometry based on the power of the tetrahedron and the spiral manifested in Layer Thirteen, representing the cosmic forces that bring closer thought and the expression of a celestial language, determining the observation and elevation of one's state of consciousness through the visual representation tied to the inner experience. The system of assembled geometric structures creates a group of stimuli and representations of colors and shapes that act on the observer as a concentrator and generator of energy offering us inspiration, waking us into levels of superior consciousness, into doorways that lead to the most sacred essence of being, permitting us to find the key that reconnects us to the Living Light, to experience and understand that we are all part of one superior Consciousness.

This mandala works by sending sensory stimuli while activating the light in all possible forms, amplifying to infinity the multidimensional possibilities and preparing the mind to be centered and expanded in the new knowledge that forms part of the infinite universal Wisdom. When we access this new level of consciousness, we engage new forms of creating from the pure Consciousness of Loving.

The circle integrates all shapes, interconnecting them into one. The center of all circles is a point, and that point is the beginning of any dimension and, so, of all manifestation. It connects us with all dimensions, and since it has no extension, it is total. It exists in everything; that is why it is perfect symbol of unity, of totality and of perfection. The center has it all, but only in potential, not in manifestation. From the circle, all shapes are born, thus it reveals itself in everything that exists. It teaches us that everything is an infinite progression based on the reflection of oneself: the mirror.

The maximum expression of the Flower of Life can be observed in the image of three spheres already introduced as Metatron's cube, which contains the tangible reality of all that is. In that form we find all the information of the universe condensed. We also find the number 13 once more. Each of the thirteen spheres describes in detail one aspect of our reality, including the current atomic structure.

Sacred geometry allows us to understand the unity of life and find the common origin of all forms in the integration of opposites that unifies duality everywhere, initiating the process of integration and oneness in consciousness.

By achieving the oneness of consciousness represented in the sphere, we begin to live in the consciousness of the multi-dimension, where we go from a lineal dimension to one unlimited access to the potentials contained in the ZPF. There we can create anything based on the pure and Crystalline consciousness that accompanies us. The multidimensional consciousness that we build from this tetrahedral perfection is mathematically constructed as a divine matrix, as a self-existing order of numerical and harmonious relations linked among themselves.

In the perfection of creation, there are no irrational or broken numbers; there are a series of fractals with infinite exponential power, allowing for the transcendence of limits in 3D and connecting to the multi-dimension.

That is why neither time nor space can be conceived as linear, because they do not have a beginning point or end point. The IRB project transforms the molecular disposition in every being, even if it is invisible, and of our material world. This new molecular disposition teaches us that we do not need conflict to grow; it activates the power of Love and Light and makes fear imperceptible. Thoughts become 100% creative, making the consciousness of instant creation whatever is appropriate in the moment. The density we experience in the current dimension becomes subtle and incorporates for each person the lesson that allows us to create from consciousness. The resulting group consciousness is unity. The individual advancement positively affects the group in a synergetic manner, and obviously the group's advancement is the individual's advancement.

Another perfect shape is the spiral. All geometric shapes previously discussed are complemented by the spiral, a geometric form that is generated by the heart when we feel love. When energy creates spiral currents (which in IRB are referred to as cones), it produces infinity, with a spiral that points down (the receptive) and points upward (the projective). The feminine spiral allows us to receive information from the cosmos; the masculine projects our energy forward to create life wherever it may find itself. The spiral unifies all geometric shapes and makes them travel in space. Therefore, every Platonic solid is a consciousness vessel. IRB, as part of its initiation process, uses these cones as symbols of the two spirals.

Two types of spirals are known: the Golden and the Fibonacci. The Golden is a cosmic spiral, such as our own galaxy, having no beginning or end.

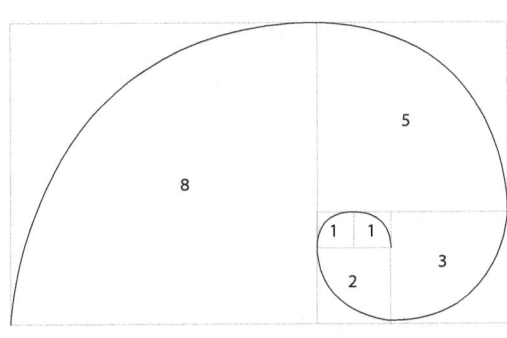

Aurea Proportion

While the Fibonacci spiral begins at a set point, which relates to the human body as part of this dimensional moment, the spiral begins in the energetic center of the heart, reaching into space and connecting with the Golden spiral and forming what Winter (2002) referred to as the toroid. The power that moves the heart is Love, and Love is the intelligence that connects us to the great Wisdom of the universe and generates an energetic toroid with an infinite amount of possibilities of combinations that become the master key to access the science of creation.

When waves self-organize into a rose-like pattern or fractal, as has been amply discussed by Winter, they give birth to all powers: life, gravity, perception, color, ecstasy and illumination, which means we can literally design sacred and healing places when we activate and become aware of these electro-fractal fields.

Through the above Dan Winter has designed revolutionary technologies to obtain hydrogen energy, purify water, heal lakes, and recharge crystals, plus heal with them, using a base in his equation for the structure of hydrogen, which is nothing more than the rose pattern previously mentioned. Winter says:

> Nature made all living proteins fractals in its construction and until we learn to build houses, hospitals and cities with the electric field geometry, we will continue to bleed fractality which is the definition of all pain.

IRB activates through initiating consciousness through the union of fractals, the toroid, and ourselves, to build this new Earth, this new reality from the OMAK.

The Fibonacci spiral is used by nature to grow. We find it in animals, plants, flowers, fruits and minerals. In the spatial layout of the Giza pyramids we also find the spiral or the Fibonacci progression. The spiral is the key to achieving the connection with the field and with DNA, which also has a spiral form.

Mantras, or sacred chants, have the inner structure of the spiral. Although supposedly, using the perception of our 3D senses, music cannot be seen by our eyes, it is totally composed of sacred geometry. This is why a mantra is always chanted repeatedly: repetition forms the spiral in space. In Chapter XVIII, we discussed how important it is to begin to listen to our DNA instead of speaking to it or giving it instructions from an obsolete belief system. We also discussed how our DNA, when spoken to, listens in alpha tones. That is why the appropriate mantras, situated beyond conscious understanding and designed under sacred tetrahedral geometry and perfectly formed spirals, are capable of taking DNA to its maximum expression of perfection, in absolute unity with OMAK, with the divine matrix.

3. The Thymus Gland

The thymus gland exerts a strong influence on the development and maturation of the lymphatic system and the immune response of the body. It also has great influence on the development of the sexual glands. It is a gland shaped like a pyramid, with a quadrangular base. It consists of two lobes, right and left, and is located behind the top of the sternum. The thymus is much more developed at birth than in adulthood. What is believed is that it grows until puberty then begins a slow involution as the gland is replaced by adipose tissue. This is basically due to the thymus gland actually being the happiness gland — and here it is very important to emphasize that happiness is not having or possessing what we desire from our thoughts or beliefs; happiness is simply being; happiness comes from acceptance. When we grow up and abandon the authenticity of our inner child, and we become adults charged with responsibilities and limitations, we leave behind our true selves, connected instead to doing and having. At that point, the thymus gland stops being nourished since it is fed by laughter and happy moments. It grows when we are happy and shrinks when we are stressed, and even more so when we are ill. This is why for a long time medicine has been confused, as only through autopsy has it been learned that the thymus had shrunken in size. It has even been said that after seven years of age this gland is reabsorbed and disappears into our bodily tissues.

The thymus produces the thymic hormone, which is very important to the functioning of the immune system. We know that it is capable of modifying the lymphocytes from the matured bone-marrow cells, the agents that immunologically respond to infectious disease.

The thymus stores fear and, along with the spleen, rules over our immune system. In a situation of panic, fear makes a person becomes smaller, and when this occurs the body allows for the entrance of viruses. When a person "gets" a virus, it is because at some point he or she felt fear or one of its manifestations. The place where we touch with our forefinger when we say "I" is where the thymus gland can be touched and stimulated. Its meaning is vital energy, and I believe that is all it needs to be, in regard to being the fundamental vessel of transformation.

Part of the manipulation to hide, or separate us from, our OMAK, has been to conceal the amazing power we have within our physical bodies, specifically as a communications hub that all calls go through, permitting connections from inner to outer.

Just like the pineal gland, the thymus gland is highly sensitive to images, lights, colors and other sensorial stimuli, as well as words and thoughts. That is why we adorn this place with Loving Jewelry, keeping our immune system efficient. Our thoughts have power over viruses and bacteria, just as thoughts of Light and Loving have power to activate all our powers.

IRB works in this change of consciousness where all is transformed into Living Loving Light, which is how this gland is activated to maximum expression through being initiated with IRB.

4. Meditation

Be that which you truly are.

For those who live in the Self as the beauty devoid of thought, there is nothing to be thought of.

The only thing we must adhere to is the experience of silence, since in this supreme state there is nothing to reach beyond our own selves.

Sri Ramana Maharshi

When a person transcends the Self, there is no more seeing, having or achieving. There is only being. Great teachers such as Osho, Maharishi, and many others who have come to this planet to generate Conscious consciousness, have spoken of this state of conscious awareness. It does not mean the achievement of some goal in our destiny. It simply means to be what we truly are and always have been, in spite of forgetting our true divine essence. All we need to do is abandon the acceptance of the illusion as our reality; to stop considering the unreal as real. When we are able to abandon this practice, it is then that we reach the OMAK, which is so self-evident and has always been available to us, though our hypnotized state has for so many years prevented us from seeing it. We will consider it a Utopia, that today when we are conscious through IRB.

For many years, certain meditations have taught us to observe the observer, and it turns out there's actually no observer observing anything. The observer overseeing everything, ceases to exist, as all there truly is, is the Self.

Maharshi also said, "Know that the many objective differences are not real but mere superimpositions on the Self, which is the form of true knowledge."

After sound, comes great silence. Silence changes the heart. In the sacred silence of our heart is where we can find the thoughts shared with a humanity long manipulated by limiting beliefs. There we can replace them with our own thoughts of Living light and Love that allow us to achieve this new shared reality, adding more focus to the hundredth monkey effect. Silence is the loudest form of prayer, the most potent initiation, and the way that allows us to go beyond words, beyond meaning, and beyond symbols. For the meditator, silence is the most eloquent instruction. It is also Grace in its highest form of expression; Grace and Divinity are the same thing. All other initiations, for example, words, looks and teachings, are derived from silence. Therefore, they are secondary yet implicit. Silence is the primary form, the most perfect one, one that understands the other initiations. If your heart achieves silence, the mind purifies itself to activate the Creator from the OMAK.

Meditations designed through IRB as part of initiation to this life project, connect us to our "within" and "without," as it is we who create the conditions that lead us within and we prepare inwardly to come to our center. Likewise, IRB pushes us from the "outside," creating attraction from "inside," allowing the human to establish him or herself from the center. In silence duality disappears, ceasing to exist. Silence is a dynamic, eternal, universal force. Allow yourself, dear reader, to be initiated in silence, with the power of the Indigo Ray in perfect balance.

Many may ask themselves: why do we need an initiation if silence is available to all? The answer to this question lies in an old story of Oriental wisdom that goes something like this:

A king visited his prime minister at the prime minister's home, where he was told the man was busy meditating, which consisted of repeating sacred syllables, or mantras. The king waited, and when the prime minister finally appeared, the king asked about the sacred words that the man had spent an hour repeating. The king was told it was the most sacred of mantras: the Gayatri. The King wished to be initiated by the prime minister, who confessed his inability to do so. The king had to learn from another person, and when, later, he saw the prime minister again, he recited the Gayatri for him, asking if he had learned it correctly. The minister replied that the mantra was correct but that it was not appropriate for the king if he was not achieving the sacred effects desired. Under the King's pressure for an explanation, the prime minister ordered a nearby servant boy to arrest the King. The servant did not obey. The command was repeated many times, but the boy did not listen. The king became angry and ordered the same servant to arrest the minister, an order which was immediately complied with. The minister laughed and said the king now had his explanation. "How...?" began the King. The minister replied, "The command was the same, and so was the person obeying the command, but not the authority. When I made the command, nothing happened.

But when you did it, there was an immediate effect. The same is true of mantras."

IRB has found a portal, and it is through this portal that we must all go to correctly access the information that tunes us into our life purpose and personal evolution. By reading this book alone, you're already on your way to finding this portal.

Meditation through IRB is different from other meditation techniques since it does not require effort, or silencing the mind, or focusing on anything specific, yet it permits our consciousness to spontaneously access this unlimited essence, expressing our potential within the conscience of unity and activating the totality of all potentials available to us naturally in the ZPF. Consciousness awakens our unlimited dignity, our inexhaustible essence, and our infinite potential. When consciousness tunes into the perfection of the OMAK within the ZPF, the amplitude of its complete existence is accepted: activity and silence, a single point and infinity. There is no need to obtain a new set of beliefs; simply remove the limitations and from a new philosophy of infinite consciousness generate a new reality. That has always been in the present and the totality, though within the limited system of beliefs that you currently have, it may seem impossible.

5. Speed

The agitated world that we participate in drives us at break-neck speed through life. We want to compete against time, gain time, consume time; we want to turn back time; we want for night to come soon so we can rest or enjoy pleasures; we want time to move faster so we can go on vacation. It is those precious moments when we believe we can truly enjoy our partners, our friends, a nice place, our family, or whatever it is. And then we want something else, something different.... Later we will discuss time versus the present moment. For now, let's just focus on the speed with which we are living, the speed and quality of our thoughts, and the attention we give each of them.

Wanting everything to happen faster, eating "fast food" and better yet watching "sixty-second news," drinking instant coffee, reacting to instant opinions.... Speed turns us into robots and keeps us from acting from love and enjoying the present moment. Is it logical that, out of the 365 days granted us by the Gregorian calendar, we can hope to enjoy only fifteen of those days in freedom? That of seven days in a week, we can only have one or two to rest? Out of twenty-four hours in the day, we can only have two or three to share with those we love? Is that the life that we want to continue to create and build? There are only two options: either we enjoy what we do twenty-four hours out of the day, 365 days of the year, or we need to find a life that produces joy in us all the time. That is why it is necessary to activate the information that IRB proposes in each of our cells.

Our experience of time has much to do with speed. When we slow down an accelerated rhythm, we can observe everything happening around us. While we live, there are millions and millions of beings, of live particles, of atoms and quarks, simultaneously living in a multi-dimension that we can experience when we become one with everything.

If we were to slap our hand carelessly across a high quality microphone, we would hear the resulting sound: loud and pointless. Now if we were to pass our hand over the same microphone in a much slower, softer, subtle way, we would be able to hear through the resulting sound everything going on in the room and even pass into a subtle state of meditation that allows us to perceive things beyond the senses. This is an example of how velocity affects us.

The same thing happens when we eat. Sometimes we don't chew but just wolf down our food, missing the combination of flavors, of temperatures, of textures, and of all the magical goodness included in each mouthful. This not only prevents us from enjoying each bite to the fullest, it also sends the food to our stomach without proper pre-digestion, leading to obesity, malnutrition, stomach issues and anxiety. Speed brings anxiety to our lives, and anxiety brings addictions.

Anxiety invites us to look for more rather than enjoy what we have. It anchors the thought of not being complete, since there is so much information we do not see due to our excessive speed. This results in our feeling empty. We fail to gather all the information in our journey, so as to reach the destination set for ourselves when we began. The pleasure is not in getting there; the pleasure is in the journey. This is found to be true in sex, food, breathing and living. Enjoyment, being happy, is directly related to the speed at which we live.

In modern dialect, one of the most pejorative words you can use for someone is "slow." The invitation from IRB is to stop purchasing or otherwise absorbing life from outside sources. Let us create it, design it, live it, enjoy it step by step. Every nanosecond there is something to feel. Let us not think it; let us simply love it; since Love is eternal, it is unhurried. Let us turn our lives, our time, our speed, into an ongoing meditation. Let us go farther, let us listen to the beyond, let us perceive each aroma and every flavor more deeply, let us feel everything experienced each moment, from the essence of the All, of infinity. Everything has been created for us so that, from this moment, we can dare go through the portal that IRB opens, and to live each scene of our existence, created for us in a positive, relaxed way looking through an exciting slow-motion camera.

Let us transcend the senses with this new speed that allows us to create true compassion, that heals from the Blue Ray, from that nearly black Indigo Ray that allows us to perceive a new spectrum of light and color that we never knew existed — not to try to understand, but simply to see that no moment is empty, that what we experience from a slower speed is unique and unrepeatable, and that every action is a meditation, because we become conscious of the presence, from the here-and-now where we all are.

One of my favorite and most recommended movies to truly understand what we are trying to express in regard to speed is the movie *Peaceful Warrior* (2006, directed by Victor Salva). To live slowly is to activate longevity, is to make love to life, is to know from the deepest part of ourselves that we are Consciousness.... The key is to live in a leisurely way from the highest, most vibrant frequencies. The combination of the two tunes us into the frequency of Love.

6. The Hologram

A considerable number of scientists (Karl Pribram, Karl Lashley, David Bohm, Stephen Hawking, Jacob D Bekenstein, Hugo Zuccarelli, Alain Aspect, Gerard't Hooft, Leonard Suskind, Craig Hogan, and Basil Hiley, among others) have discussed, experienced and analyzed the concept of the hologram.

For example, Alain Aspect, along with an important team of researchers, discovered that in certain circumstances subatomic particles such as electrons are capable of communicating instantly with others, no matter the distance that separates them. It doesn't matter if this distance is one foot or hundreds of thousands of miles. Without exception, one particle knows what the other is doing. If we explore deeper into this, it means that thought travels faster than light. Einstein established that no communication travels faster than the speed of light. Yet the new reality disproves that old principle.

On the other hand, Einstein's disciple, David Bohm, considered Aspect's discoveries an indication that objective reality does not exist; despite the apparent solidity of mass, the universe is actually an enormous, fantastic hologram filled in with incredible detail. The nature of "the whole in every part" aspect of the hologram allows for an entirely new way of understanding the whole system. Bohm suggests that what empowers distant particles to remain in contact with each other despite the distance separating them, is not some kind of mysterious signal but simply the fact that separation is an illusion. Bohm suggests that, at a deeper level of reality, these particles are not individual entities but extensions of the same fundamental thing.

To better explain what he means, Bohm offers the following illustration:

> Imagine an aquarium containing a fish. Imagine also that you cannot see this aquarium directly and your only knowledge of the aquarium is due to two recording cameras, one pointed at the front and the other at the side. When you watch the two monitors, you end up believing the fish on each screen is an individual entity. This is because the cameras are pointed at different angles, so each image is slightly different. But if you continue to watch the two fish, you end up becoming aware that there is a relationship between the two. When one turns, the other turns, as well, if slightly differently. When one turns to face the front, the other turns to face the side. If you don't know about the angles of the cameras and you let yourself be guided by your senses, you will reach the conclusion that the two fish are communicating, despite it clearly not being the case.

According to Bohm:

> Currently, the fastest connection to life is apparently subatomic particles, telling us that there exists a deeper level of reality that we are part of, the more complex dimension beyond our own dimension which is similar to the fish in the aquarium.

He adds:

> We see objects such as these subatomic particles as if they were separated from others because we are only seeing a part of them. The apparent separation of the subatomic particles is an illusion; this means that it is through love that everything in the universe is infinitely interconnected.

In a holographic universe such as the one we live in, even time and space cannot be seen in a radical fashion, since concepts such as location are shattered with the new perspective that nothing is truly separate, since time and space are multidimensional. Just like the images of the fish on the monitors, our "reality" can be seen as a magically profound projection, like a super hologram in which the past, present and future exist simultaneously. We could even say the great hologram is the matrix that gave birth to everything in our universe, so therefore it contains every subatomic particle of everything that is. If this material world that we can observe and touch with each of our senses is nothing more than a secondary reality, what we believe to be real is nothing more than optical or sensorial illusion created by holographic frequencies. And if the brain is the medium through which we select some of the frequencies of this illusion to mathematically transform into something that we believe to be real, then what is reality?

A hologram, to explain it in a simpler way, is like a photograph that contains all the dates and general characteristics of the photographed object or subject; therefore, it contains all that's necessary for observation in three dimensions. A hologram is produced when a single laser light is split into two separate beams. The first beam is bounced off the object to be photographed. The second beam is allowed to collide with the reflected light of the first. When this happens they create an interference pattern that is then recorded on film. If that image, let's say of an apple, is then cut in half and illuminated by a laser, each half will still be found to contain the entire image of the apple! Even if the halves are divided again and again, an entire apple can still be seen in each portion of the photo (though the images will get hazier as the portions become smaller). Unlike normal photographs, every small fragment of a piece of holographic film contains all the information recorded in the whole.

One of the possibilities brought forth by the hologram is that, if the angle at which the two lasers reach a piece of the exposed film is changed, it is possible to record different registries on the same surface. Therefore, if the universe possesses this holographic characteristic, everything we may perceive in the astral planes and the domains of the angels, is simply another "registry angle." According to each person's synchronization, the angle of our registry may vary, in this way permitting each of us to create our own holographic universe by means of our angle of view, allowing each of us to observe the same registry in a different way.

We can consciously use the "reading laser" we each possess in this 3D world, as can potentially the whole world. We activate or, better, calibrate this consciousness tool by activating the OMAK. We can modify the hologram of our universe at any angle necessary to see it and read it in a way that is appropriate to our individual consciousness, permitting us to navigate through mental multidimensionality, and even physically, since the physical is only a projection of the mental. This confirms the concepts of Carl Jung, who said that everything we call reality is part of a collective unconscious shared by all people.

To understand the concept of the hologram, so common in today's electronics, is to arrive at the concept that we are reflections of what we project, conscious or unconsciously, about ourselves. Even the apparent physical structure of the body is the holographic projection of the consciousness. If we take this to the level of "healing" (when we talk about paradigms, we'll go more into depth on this concept), we will understand the truth behind what we call miracles, which is nothing more than instant communication between subatomic particles that allows us to create new points of life in our reality.

In the 1990s, physicists Leonard Susskind and Gerard 't Hooft confirmed that the theory of a holographic universe has the same importance as the theory of relativity, or quantum medicine, or string theory, since it is not just someone's abstract idea with complex concepts but a theory that comes from a new interpretation of long-accepted scientific concepts.

Therefore, we can conclude that we know our external reality through our senses. When we observe an object or a physical manifestation, what we do is interpret the reception of light photons through the eye into the brain, then the brain is in charge of putting together a three-dimensional image based on electrochemical impulses. We never participate in this reality-construction in a direct manner, as we barely understand how we perceive our surrounding and ourselves. Meaning, that which we call exterior reality, is actually not outside but inside our brain because that is how we create it. To think that what we see or touch is real, is an illusion formed by codified signals from the brain.

When every human is equipped with the same mechanisms and, from birth, conditioned to see a manipulated outer reality, we share many impressions in common and end up believing that we are living in a "proven" material world. A movie that clearly illustrates this theory is The Hunger Games series (based on the novels of Suzanne Collins, from 2008).

Therefore, if the entire universe is a hologram, and the surroundings that we perceive is a reality we are only imagining, we can re-create and co-create differently from our new connection to Consciousness with all the power of the OMAK offered to us by IRB.

7. The Mantras

In principle, and in a very basic way, mantras are syllables, words or groups of words, whose aim is to achieve a level of concentration that frees the creative mind. The most ancient and world-renowned mantras were designed in Sanskrit and used for mental or verbal repetition. The point is not to know the meaning behind what is being said or sung, so as not to fill the mind with specific thoughts, but instead a means of empty the mind and in this way getting to our center and finding peace and tranquility there. The rhythm and vibration mantras produce have the power to cause great internal changes. When we chant a mantra, the mind has no time for other thoughts; therefore, we achieve a state of deep relaxation and meditation.

The basic concept of mantras is the architecture of sound, the vibration and the energy generated by the vibration, which tunes us into a specific frequency; from there they have the ability to generate changes in the field in which they are being sung and within the person singing them. If we stopped to fully and consciously listen to our surroundings, we would surprise ourselves with the variety of ways sound can be produced. Every movement, for example, is an expression of sound that we may or may not be able to hear with our ears. But even in the most profound of silences, there is sound, though we may not always be aware of it. Some sounds have resonance with others. The sacred language that originates from silence is unique and universal. The vibration we receive from silence transcends all limits, showing us that, despite all the differences in form, we all come from the same Source. Each of us is a fundamental instrument in the grand orchestra of the universe, to be lived and manifest.

The vibration that a mantra provides permits us to install a new model that totally restores, revitalizes and reorders our energy systems, connecting them to more subtle frequencies. When we elevate the vibrational octaves of our cells, we open the door into expanded Consciousness, with which we are able to experience the invisible or subconscious world in a more real way, which consciously affects our hologram. It is said at the correct repetition of the mantras channeled by IRB leads us to recognize ourselves and act in Loving Truth, Living Light Vision, Wisdom, Presence and Compassion, all from the totality that unites us with Oneness.

Sound is a powerful stimulus that affects cell function, creating the necessary conditions for reestablishment of the OMAK. Mantras and music manifested through IRB generate field-conscious electromagnetic waves that interact with the organism, deeply penetrating it, reaching the nucleus of information in the cells, producing the activation of the Nuclear Commands that give life to Layer Thirteen of our DNA. This launches the symphony that every being is prepared to perform in their lives.

As was previously explained, our first vehicle of transformation, the pineal gland, is intimately linked to this and all the rest, both the music and the mantras manifested for the activation of all the transformation vessels of IRB, are based on the 1-1-0 Key, which Hurtak explains in detail in The Book of Knowledge: The Keys of Enoch: "The key languages that connect the distortions of time-mind to interconnected civilizations and manifestations of 'superior evolution' in our zone-time are: Egyptian-Hebrew-Sanskrit-Tibetan-Chinese[…]"

This key explains that ,if we interconnect with these five sacred languages, we will mentally interconnect with civilizations that represent "superior evolution." Therefore, IRB activates the four

Nuclear Commands with energetic sacred sounds and thought-forms of light to make the connection with the intelligences of superior planes, unifying all the crystalline languages that open the blueprint of the mind to the Eternal and Living Light. This permits activation of pictographic communication of the highest universal frequencies in the brain, thus creating a mental distortion of time that vivifies the OMAK of human recipients of the experience of consciousness, through the cosmic light vibration that unifies the totality of the being within his or her most supreme essence.

Here these sounds are transformed into a language of energetic vibration formed by carefully selected seed mantras. These vibrations raise the corporal consciousness to the seed-crystalline mind, setting our consciousness paradigm off on a spiral trajectory. We can enter this dimension where all life movement becomes eternal unfoldment, where everything is lived and recycled because the universe has every idea stored in the eternal mind of reflection and revelation. We can access any dimension using this light-point through the ZPF.

These mantras are provided in the first level of initiation into IRB, to be able to obtain the appropriate vibration when crossing the doorway to the consciousness of our own self-creation.

To get a little closer to what the thirteen mantras do within us, we're going to give a brief description of each.

The first four (clarifying that "first" does not correspond to the linear order established in this 3D world) are activated through one of the Nuclear Command. Later we will explain what we mean by the four Nuclear Commands that activate the 1-1-0 Key, which has already been introduced. They are supported by the energy of Loving, to activate the totality of what is, in sacred quantum DNA:

NETZACH MERKAVA ELIYAHU: The first mantra is in charge of activating the first three layers, supporting the evolution of incarnation and accessing the multi-dimension.

EHYEH ASHER EHYEH: The second mantra is in charge of activating the second three layers, developing the power of manifestation from the inner Christ, from the reflection of the sacredness manifested on Earth.

SHECHINAH-ESH: The third is in charge of the next three layers, including learning of all our experiences, lived and yet to be lived, from the power of transformation and a change of perspective toward a new reality.

EL SHADAI: The fourth is in charge of activating the third and fourth layers that manifest most sacred Divinity, incorporating all of the Light Beings in our DNA, so that we may live from the point of view of who we truly are in our Divine Origin.

Together these four mantras, combined with the music and frequency of IRB from the first Nuclear Command, allow us to open ourselves to the frequency of Infinite Loving in our reality.

The next five activate the second of the four Nuclear Commands, which allow us to recognize the Truth, speak in Truth, and live within it being conscious of each act and manifestation created.

AMEN PTAH: The fifth mantra is in charge of activating the inner masculine, with so much strength that it permits that all of the power of action, from full Wisdom and Presence, become a part of daily life. It is the same overwhelming loving order that opens the cave hiding the greatest treasures available to us in any existing dimension.

GABRIEL: The sixth has the power of transferring divine power with the spoken word. It opens the ability to speak from absolute and creative Truth, sustaining the pure and the diaphanous in the verb of creation itself. It is androgyny, which completes it in the most delicate of balances within the recognition of power and action, and always within the grand frame of humility.

BUDDAH: The power of transmission of the seventh mantra in the second Nuclear Commands is so powerful that it makes practical application of well-being as it relates to Oneness from the All. This mantra generates absolute understanding that nothing is separate, that nothing exists independently, whether atoms, people or cultures. Thus it activates altruism from Knowing, unifying spirituality and science. It permits us to understand that the physical body, our image, our bank account, is a simple phenomenon, a matter of appearance that we have given meaning and value that we lack in ourselves. It ends the mind-games that create the significance and labels we attribute to objects. Meaning, it frees us from ignorance, from the "I," and connects us with the All. It permits us to update the information from the everyday mind to the universal, unified mind, where everything is interconnected; accessing a new form of perceiving reality, changing the station that we have tuned into up until now to the "real world" and establish ourselves in the world of Consciousness, of spirit, of science and art yet to be explained. A new reality is created in accord with this new Balanced Consciousness, Living Light and Love, that permits us to act in accordance with being a wave vibrating at high frequencies, within which we can navigate through diverse dimensions. This is not only for elevated mathematicians, physicists or renowned spiritual leaders; it is for you and me, for all who wish to have an existential leap in their consciousness in a daily and permanent way. It requires neither explanations nor scientific demonstrations; nor do we need to know how it works. It is simply necessary to put it into effect, the same way that we do not need to know all the mechanical details of a car in order to drive.

PHOWA: The eighth mantra transfers consciousness at the moment of death, as we go through the bardo of enlightenment, where we truly understand the greatness of our spirits, beyond our bodies and minds. It confers the ability to illuminate everything surrounding us, permitting the mind to remain in a permanent state of pleasure in a new reality in which ego and illusion are no longer the Masters of life. Timeless Presence takes precedence in our quantum transformation. At this moment, any hint of fear is transmuted into the energy of Learning.

KWAN YIN: The ninth complements the inner masculine with the feminine deity that activates in our being, special codes of mercy and fortune, permitting us to assimilate each creative sound in our personal universe. As a fundamental part of this tool, it is also in charge of activating Compassion, which permits us to remain in a quantum state of healing, which leads to living in absolute freedom. The ninth mantra activates the power of the mirror, the power to reflect back to the entire universe from the heart of essential Wisdom; it possesses the beat of life that always brings life. It completely opens our ability to hear the great sound of silence that is the absolute sound of the divine voice, permitting us to be One with all that surrounds us. This mantra has the ability to make the cells tune into the part of the ZPF where vitality and youth, joined with the masculine and feminine, reflect the transformation of balance in the human life and in the planet we represent. It is the Ray of Compassion in action that contains the great ocean of creation from original Consciousness, visible to the highest levels of light destined for us and our creation apart from duality.

LAY-OO-ESH: The tenth mantra activates the third Nuclear command in charge of amplifying the vision and projecting the Living Light that is God in action.

This mantra is so potent that it acts directly, without help from anything else, on one of the Nuclear Commands. It is the spark that ignites the fire of creation. There is no further explanation required. Is a great sign provided to us as part of the IRB project, that permits the crowning of the pyramid in the light of Christ from the highest spheres. It now comes to us on the pyramidal bases of the crystal field Urim and Tumim, here on this sacred Earth, our beloved indigo planet, and it connects us to the reality that we are part of God's people. Not like a religion or dogma, but as part of a mission. By activating the tenth mantra, all mysteries are revealed, so the pyramid will not have such a great distance between the point and the base (read The Biggest Secret, 1998) and we will all be part of the "all seeing eye," including the wonders of eternity. This activation merges us with the Pillar of light that rests in the tabernacle on the journey to the next level of creator intelligence.

To activate this fourth Nuclear Command, which is in charge of the supreme connection to Superior Wisdom, we have been given three mantras. None of the thirteen mantras are anything new; they have always been here, visible yet veiled. Only now they are here with the intention of quantum awakening of their greatness. Not greatness within ego, but as the magnificence of who we truly are.

SHEM HA MEPHORASH: The first mantra of this command, the eleventh, is the un-manifested cosmic principle. It contains creation in itself. This mantra has been hidden for years in the book of Exodus in the Hebrew Bible and is made up by all of God's names, which were applied to God so no one would call him by his true name, which was said to be unspeakable. In Layer Thirteen of our DNA, we will also find the director that orchestrates creation from Loving, Presence, Compassion and Wisdom. It permits us to turn into salvation itself and for our name to be written in eternity. By becoming a mantra of activation for this important Nuclear Command, with its appropriate initiation, it begins to be a part of this rebirth in the new quantum vibration of our DNA and opens way for the final two. This is why, despite containing the power of 13 within it, the power that activates IRB is 11.

YOD HE VAU HE: The second mantra in this command, the twelfth, contains the power of the Tetragrammaton, released by the brotherhoods of the Old World as a symbol of power. This mantra was hidden for years and misrepresented by many as a means for manipulation. Now from this new energy it gives us the sacred base of the fourth that, along with sacred geometry, gives life, as noted in the paragraph on the tetrahedron. Human life is created from this mantra. The zygote, when divided, generates a tetrahedron in its base structure, from which all perfection is created, which later self-generates in the maternal womb. It is associated with the heart, as Nuclear Command of Creation, of Love. It works together with what came before, containing the ineffable name that gives life to all sublime creation from eternal Living Light. When we activate the codes of light contained in these four letters, we can self-generate from Love and the eternal Living Light of the creator which we have called God to avoid using his true name.

KADOSH, KADOSH, KADOSH, ADONAI TSEBAYOTH: The last mantra, the thirteenth, as part of the activation of this Nuclear Command, unifies what we have called negativity in the dense body of this dimension, creating bridges to other dimensions and activating the sacred grids of our bodies. This is a bridge in the 3D world to other dimensions. When we dwell in this song we become of one heart, joining the inferior levels of vibration with the highest levels of creation, which permits the circulatory system to incorporate the beat of the cosmic heart, as it establishes a connection among all hierarchies. The energy of light created by this sacred name prepares the body to experience energy directly from the Masters of light, who become part of us. This mantra contains additional scales of chromatic resonance, emanating eighty octaves above and eighty octaves below our planet. This sacred code connects to the infinite, balancing all that is positive and negative as a single creative force, as it activates the special grids of harmonic resonance with the brotherhood of light and permits energy to join together for mutual work and worship. This Nuclear Command, along with IRB, combines with music and frequency manifested for this tool, a hyper vortex or pillar of divine energy through which space-time travels to put us in resonance with other levels of divine intelligence.

This is why, being thirteenth, it completes the sequence.

8. Nuclear Commands

Key 1-0-6 in Hurtak's previously referenced book tells us that our universe was created from a "Synthesis of Light" as the cradle and throne of our consciousness. To be able to sit on this throne, it is important to calibrate our being, and for this we need the four Nuclear Commands that activate the vehicles of transformation, to access the OMAK from our nucleus. The activation of these Nuclear Commands takes us to the center, to the nuclear energy that molds the atomic nucleus that is then used in building the physio-energetic system of our visible galaxy, to use it as a purifier of light still caught up in the old energy. The activation of those Nuclear Commands represents the key to new creation on this physical plane, the galactic principle of the physical Adamic family.

Below is a message from Kryon channeled through Marina Mecheva, especially for IRB in the beginning of the year 2013 when this project began:

> [...] It has to do with personal calibration. This is what you will use to move before you complete this, so that you can take it to a higher level. Allow us to continue to complete this exchange sharing with you an open heart, and open throat chakra, and open third eye, and an open crown. They are to anchor the reality through the three inferior energetic centers. You are moving through a synchronicity that deals with the centers particularly, to allow healing, releasing calibration of the Self in a new way; by moving through these models of your own reality, of your own behavior and your own being, there will be a sense of lightness that will come from a much higher place...
>
> [...] All this has to do with the system that is developing. For your mission is to help others remember their purest self and to achieve this, you must help them reach a place where they feel lighter and where they have left enough space available for their superior Self to enter [...]
>
> [...] This is what you are working toward, empowering others through your empowerment. We salute you from inside, while we begin the movement toward the energy dynamic that is ready to go to the next level. Continue, continue and don't stop, for what moves you inside is the engine of inspired love, inspired love, and so it is."

When these words reached us, we were already trying out these Nuclear Commands. According to what was given to us, it is not necessary to activate each individual particle, since previous work has tuned up the vehicle. All that is required is to turn it on, and it can take flight and fulfill its ultimate divine purpose in this current state of consciousness.

There are no limits. There is only the beginning of the next 26,000 years, to be populated by the Indigo Race, the Seventh Race, as witnesses to the nations in evolution. This race Hurtak refers to as beings with the spiritual power of the Christ that are also incorporated by IRB into this consciousness of superior light. The effect is similar to a hotbed or the cradle nurturing and sustaining this pre-existing consciousness of light. The cradle is where the seed of consciousness passes into the physical matrix of space and time, through the chosen ones, opening the opportunity for those answering the call to graduate to superior universes, understanding that "the chosen" does not refer to one, but to all; it is about self-election. The possibilities exist for all, free will never being restricted; thus we are always free to choose.

These four Nuclear Commandments are considered fundamental to the harmony of creation, as they allow those who listen to the call to go through their activation, purifying their thoughts and energy, and reaching the state of "divine no-evolution" (to transcend it rather than requiring it), which qualifies them to dress the body of the OMAK, giving them the knowledge to endow all species with the ability to bring light to other creations in unison. Together, we can go through this great doorway that elevates us to the level of superior stellar intelligences, as one single family united in divinity, completely free.

The four Commandments activate our nuclear energy, opening the skies by removing the control handle and permitting us to tune into the true stellar indicator of superior planes in perfect harmony. Thoughts of war and destruction will no longer occur; there is only Living Light and Loving within the OMAK, whose codes are accessible to all. In this way, the Nuclear Commands offer us the keys necessary to put into action the program of freedom against the lineal forces of Babylonian control that have enslaved us to render homage to the inferior heavens for eons. This permits us to purify our vehicle to such a point that our self-mastery generates the power to materialize new heavens on this Earth, from infinite gematria that sets us free.

The Four commandments are:

1. The Heart Command
2. The Throat Command
3. The Third Eye Command
4. The Crown Command

In the second CD of the music album Activación Divina (Divine Activation), simultaneously channeled along with this same information, we have the thirteen mantras, divided by the commands to which they pertain.

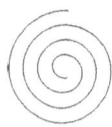

Chapter XXI
The Concepts

Our heads are round so our thoughts can change direction.
Francis Picabia

1. Infinity

Infinity, as the name indicates, has an endless number of meanings. It is almost impossible to explain infinity with the limited human language, since infinity is of a purely quantum nature. To have a better grasp of this concept that immerses us in the totality and beyond possibilities, it is important to understand what infinity is not: it is not linear, it has no limits, no beginning and no end, and it transcends both the alpha and the omega. IRB has a pure quantum connection with the Essence, with the ALL, with the Consciousness of Being — of being "I" and being the universe, in the here and now, in the vacuum whose name is Infinity.

The closest it comes to our weak concept of infinity lies a quote from T.S. Elliot. When referring to the universe, Elliot asked himself how it was possible that something could come from nothing: "Or say that the end precedes the beginning, and the end and the beginning were always there, before the beginning and after the end. And all is always now."

As we have amply explained and will continue to, we exist in a universe that rests on possibilities and not absolutes. Binary philosophy, which is continually planting us in duality to show us that something either is or is not, has proven its limitations in understanding the universe. That is the reason for our fall into polarization and the war of the extremes that, thanks to quantum physics, is quickly losing ground to a perspective whereby reality is based on pulses that emit possibilities, not on definitive laws and rules.

Infinity resembles eternity, the immaterial. The known symbol that contains it, the number 8 (a sideways ∞, sometimes called the lemniscate) demonstrates an infinity dance in perfect balance, where Love vivifies in a constant give and take. It is the pure manifestation of the ZPF where everything is created in a central, neutral place; it contains *per se* all nuclear energy because everything is created from the nucleus. Everything originates from the center; everything originates from us. It harmonizes with Everything That Is in a cosmic dance that has no beginning and no end, nor does it have space or time. It just IS, in the same way we cannot determine where air begins or ends.

Infinity reminds us of the swift flight of the dragonfly, which represents the liberation of any belief that tells us we cannot do this or that, reach a goal or make a dream come true. Reminding us that everything is possible when we come to understand that we are part of Spirit, and as such have the power to manifest anything in an infinite way from infinite consciousness.

We also have the Ouroboros as an emblem of infinity. This symbol depicts the serpent eating its own tail. After eating itself, it is then reborn in infinite Consciousness, to remind us that by becoming a circle, we enter a world without limitations, where "up" and "down" are not separate opposites. All the virtues, riches and powers of your superior self transmute your physical self.

Superior and inferior fuse into one, and man (not as a gender but as a human being) becomes Divinity.

2. The Mirror

There is a story of a young man who wanted to change the world. During the prime years of his life, he preached his philosophy and his truth, but he eventually realized that his efforts had been in vain. He then decided not to continue preaching around the world but would preach only in his country, where everyone spoke the same language and would understand him better; besides, he thought, if he managed to change his country, he would also be changing the world. In the following years, the young man traveled across his country, and he got the same results. All his efforts to change things were futile. He thought it over and decided that he would begin with the city where he was born since he knew the customs and beliefs. Once he had changed his city, he decided, his country would change and then the world. So this man, now an adult, traveled his city, believing that everyone would follow. But the result was equally negative. Now an old man, he reflected on his life, thinking that he had been wrong, that he should have begun with his family. Once he changed his family, he reasoned, his city would change, then the country and lastly the world. He spent his remaining years trying to change the people closest to him, with the same results: the change never generated. On his deathbed, the man had this epyphany: "If I had only begun with myself, I could have reflected the change in my family and, in turn, my family would have reflected the change to the city, the city to the country, and the country to the world."

The universe is the reality created by each of us, and like a mirror it is always reflecting our internal conditions.

The increase in self-awareness generates evolution; it creates exponential growth that will augment our ability to observe ourselves directly, and as reflections of others. The capacity for self-observation increases our ability to know ourselves more and more, and to recognize ourselves in the reality created by others. When we reflect ourselves in others, a door opens to give us insight into ourselves, because the other is always reflecting something we cannot see or could never previously see in ourselves. When we delve in the awareness of who we are, it is similar to polishing a universal mirror in which we see ourselves, so that life reflects back infinitely, each time with greater clarity, the current manifestation of this human experience.

The more we evolve, the more vulnerable we become to internal and external triggers, for when we integrate permanently, the forms in our unconscious begin to appear, as if the entire cosmos were happening within us. At the same time, it becomes harder to distance ourselves from others because we are assuming responsibility, not only for our thoughts, words, emotions and actions, but also for those of others — through connection with ourselves — so that everything that happens lands at our own doorstep. Carl Jung operated from the maxim, "Everything that irritates us about others can lead us to an understanding of ourselves."

The fundamental concept of IRB is an example: the transformation of our personal universe as a result of our own transformation. David Icke has an analogy that I love, and which I am always sharing, having to do with wanting to comb the hair of the reflection in the mirror. If we do not like something we see reflected in the mirror, we must change it in ourselves right away, because it is impossible to change it in the reflection. This is the power to create (i.e., change) in ourselves and the ability to contribute to other's creations. It is related to the example of the flight attendant. She instructs that in case of an accident, we must first place the oxygen mask on ourselves before we even attempt to help others; it is also related to the example of Jesus, who said that he could only give what he had, even if what he possessed was only sorrow.

The principles of correspondence are simple: as above, so below; as within, so without. We cannot find anything outside of ourselves that we have not previously seen within ourselves; we cannot receive something we have not given; there cannot be a reflection of something that doesn't exist within us. There are no victims of circumstances. In the words of Aldous Huxley: "Experience is not what happens to a man; it is what a man does with what happens to him." Here comes the willingness to accept responsibility for who we are and what we think, say and do. Nothing happens by itself. We can continue being passive characters in the story, groaning and complaining, or we can begin to resonate from our own center, with the intimate frequency of our being. For this, it is important to think with the heart and to know what it is we wish to create (i.e., change) in ourselves.

The mirror is a reflection of infinity; the two create themselves together and are inseparable. When we place one mirror in front of another mirror, and we situate ourselves between them, our reflection immediately multiplies an infinite number of times. It would be impossible for each reflection to be different, for everything is created in the exact image of the original Source, which is still "ourselves" in the midst of this creation.

3. Numerology and the Alpha-Beta

Numerology is a supremely vast topic having to do with mathematics, structures, measurements, bases and science. In short, there is hardly anything in existence that doesn't contain a number. What is of interest to us here with IRB is the understanding that even letters, sounds and colors are based on numbers.

Numerology is a tool that can help us gain awareness of the structure of what we see so that we can lose identification with it and realize that our origins are absolute perfection. We can only change what we can identify; therefore, numerology brings awareness of how to change what we know.

We have already given some attention to the importance of language in the creation of mantras, and we know the name of each of our DNA layers, as given by Kryon through the Hebrew alphabet. According to Kryon, "The literal meaning of the Hebrew names is not essential for understanding the names of the DNA layers, and in some cases the Hebrew meanings are different." It means that the Hebrew language is the core language of Earth, and each name is meant to be heard as a spoken phrase, strung together for the full meaning in Hebrew. Kryon adds, "The meaning of the spoken Hebrew word lies in its energy, and therefore these Hebrew names should be spoken or heard as intended in Hebrew."

The Hebrew letters are not just tools; each letter encompasses a different type of light and a different type of energy, and each contains a number and even a color. Each DNA strand, each layer, has its own weaving characteristic, and that vibration was once encoded into the Hebrew letters. The Hebrew alphabet is a set of twenty-two letters: the three Mother letters associated with air, water and fire; the seven Double letters representing the ancient planets; and the twelve Simple letters symbolizing the twelve sectors of the celestial band traversed by the sun, the moon and the planets. We can clearly see that that these twenty-two letters summarize a macrocosmic weave and thus are the key to connecting with the strands we wish to contact.

As was said before, our interest in this case is focused on the DNA layers; each has a name in Hebrew with its corresponding letters. The combinations, given in the form of letters, can also be perceived through color and sound. The music of IRB was composed and channeled based on the structure of the notes and colors, assigning this powerful information to each element and planet.

For more than 4,000 years, we have contemplated the notion that the world is composed from a code, a language that can be articulated through a form, a number or a syllable. The syllable is the loom on which anything is woven — even the invisible, the essence. Everything is formed by the aggregation of numbers between the sound molecules. Roberto Calasso, Italian author and editor, wrote the following mysterious passage: "What to man is a number, to the gods is a syllable."

We are going to touch briefly on the meaning of numbers in this new energy. What we must understand first is that there are no negative or positive numbers, nor better numbers and worse ones. As we have stated throughout this book, there is no such a thing as "good" or "bad," and the same applies to numbers; they simply are. There is a way to interact with numbers without making them better or worse. Everything is energy and we, as co-creators of our reality, give the numbers the intention with which to function in the new co-creative universe.

IRB transcends the vibration of 33, settling on the energy of 44, which allows it to develop in the sacred symbol of infinity, the number 8. It contains the number 13, as well as 58; if we add the digits of 58, we return to 13.

The energy of 33 is the trinity, the holiness within all of your choices. Your body, mind and spirit are in perfect agreement with your Soul's evolution. Within this number, there is no indecision.

The activation of the DNA sequence gives access to the essence of Light. We are faced with that which represents light, dark matter and gray matter, without instructions, without negation and without being able to escape the truth. The number 33 places us in the consciousness of renouncement, empowering us to give up what we must.

The numerical vibration of 333 is 9, which means cosmic and personal culmination, moving to the next level of Love, Heart, and Spirit, and being at the service of planetary evolution through self-healing. The 9 also means an automatic climb to the next level of Light; a quantum leap to receiving unknown gifts.

With the essence of 44 and 13, we build a future thought-by-thought, brick-by-brick, allowing the movement of change while we remain in perfect balance with what we know to be divine truth, solidifying the platform of Light. The master number 44 takes us to the completion of a cycle and toward the infinity of the 8. With the vibration of 8, we enter the place where creation unifies the polarities ("as above so below"). This configuration gives us access to the portal of Infinity, taking us beyond the limitations we have believed in until now. It is a number that goes beyond what we know. It is pure atomic spiritual energy.

IRB opens a portal in the shape of a golden tetrahedron of power, a portal that remains open until we reach the starting point that lies in the truth of our being, the creator of instant manifestation, leaving behind the manifestations created by limitation and entering a place of crystalline creation. Doorways open and close, and we are in the middle of All. Conscious creation with thirteen-second intervals of thought. We become one with the highest essence of our being in abundant creation from the heart. All of heaven, the known and the unknown, enter through this portal. With a heart free of baggage, definitions and paradigms, we tune into the only thing that is real and true: Love.

The sound of number 13 is the sound of everything natural. There is nothing more natural than silence, which connects us to the heart and the inner universe, to the rush of our blood, the beat of our heart and the sound of our breath, turning everything into music. The Indigo area leads to neutral gray, which asks us to come in. The gray invites us to sit down and rest. The gray area is neutral, free of commentaries, pressures and stresses. We exist in multiple dimensions, and we are a central point, an intersection of currents and dimensional experiences that influence other stellar and cellular experiences. The number 1 is a singularity within the "All That Is." The 1 searches for itself in the mirror as a reflection of the world that surrounds it. The number 1 together with 3 (13) offers the opportunity to overcome any limitation we may have imposed without knowing. The 13 let us enter the Oversoul concealed in the recesses of our being, the ZPF. We don't have to fill this place, the center of our being, with thoughts of wants and needs because it represents the "vacuum" of everything that we are; here we find divine plenitude and conclusion, leaving needs behind us. It is similar to emptying a glass that is filled to the brim. When something is filled and complete, the next step is to empty it; then it can be filled again, and so on.

As was said before, everything on Earth and in the universe is defined by a numerical configuration. All life can be reduced to, and explained by, numbers. The currents of these numerical sequences bring into alignment a series of new understandings that help adjust and balance the human creature. The numbers on all levels align the body so it is able to handle the higher frequencies of photon light. Each number infusion is personalized to fit the needs of each individual, allowing them the necessary ratio of light particles to numerical particles. As the brain adjusts to these new energies, a lifting occurs allowing the individual to be lifted to the OMAK equation. Numbers and humans go hand in hand. From the beginning of time, we have been defined by a numerical equation, including age, birth date, weight, and many others.

In your daily lives, when you experience the numerical series time and again, stop for a moment and allow this energy to be birthed through you. This is the time to manifest. Each and every number in your personal universe is triggering your subconscious into a new pattern of DNA configurations.

Each of the IRB mantras is associated with a different numerical combination. We will briefly explain each number and sequence separately. It is important to tune into each number in the context of the new energy and to put aside anynegative beliefs that the old energy attached to some of them and change the connotation that kept us away from the divine truth where everything is Love.

0 and its sequences: This is the great void, what is about to be created but is not yet born. It contains everything, leading us to higher dimensions and changing our limiting perceptions about time. This is the portal of creation, containing creation within itself. It is the vibration of the absolute that allows us to be consciousness fusing with the universe. It is the center where Zero Point is manifested, where creation is possible, as it holds everything and loves unconditionally, with perfect neutrality. It is an intrinsic mandala that let us experience it from within, permitting us to fill ourselves yet empty ourselves like a universal cosmic clock.

1 and its sequences: The portal to the All. Accompanied by itself (the 11) it gives the opportunity to awaken mastery and become true light. The number 11 is the number of the masters (Kryon, for example, carries the number 11 in his essence). 11:11 on a clock is a coded molecular structure that activates our mastery — the masters have always said we are of light. When we see 11:11, at that precise moment, let us stop and become aware of our thoughts, of our creative powers; at that moment, let us join totality.

2 and its sequences: 2 stands for the most elevated sequence of creation in perfect balance. All words, thoughts, acts and intentions send down roots and grow. It allows us to welcome opposites, with no more opposing polarities, understanding that in our purest essence we are all complete. Let us set aside the old concepts of duality and doubt.

3 and its sequences: This is the number of the Trinity, which is activated within the tetrahedron in the structure of DNA. We have already spoken of this number that facilitates connection with highly evolved spiritual beings — Masters, Angels—who are not separate but part of our essence; they are a manifestation in a superior dimension — and with our inner Christ. 3 is the most powerful and impeccable antenna of communication.

4 and its sequences: This is the foundation of the eternal Living Light. It opens all possibilities. 4 is the manifestation in the density of Earth. It is the wand that, from the highest essence of our being, makes visible the highest potentials of light to manifest here and now.

5 and its sequences: 5 is the manifestation of movement and change. It enables vision by opening the eye of the mind. It is the sacred structure of our pineal gland.

6 and its sequences: For eons the vibration of the number 6 has been reviled and associated with "the beast." In this new energy of Love, where everything is welcomed and revered, number 6 connects us to the Earth and its abundance. Number 6 permits us to honor Gaia and tune into her true essence through gentleness and harmony, by turning each of our steps into a sacred path that creates a new construction for all of humanity.

7 and its sequences: I can tell you the depth and breadth of this number since I am "a seven" due to all the edges of my geometry and mathematics, both in the old and new energies. Seven is the vibration of the, of the spiritual creator. Seven works for the light, by the light, and with the light. Those of us who are seven eat, drink, think, and speak lightly. Those of us who resonate in the frequency of the number seven cannot wander beyond the limits of the light for even a second. The number seven brings us home to that place where miracles are an everyday occurrence, where we can fly and dance in the stars irrespective of the form we have manifested. The number seven, more than a number, is a place where wonder, magic, and miracles are seen as natural events. The number seven is the natural state of the being.

8 and its sequences: Another number associated intimately with IRB, 8 and its vibration open the portal to the Infinite, transporting us beyond any limitation. It is a number that allows us to fly, a spiritual atomic energy, the pure source of energy. 8 is success and prosperity. It is pure attunement with our divine heritage. It is a quantum path that, no matter the direction, permits us to savor universal abundance.

9 and its sequences: 9 is the number of rebirth, of mastery, the highest of the individual numbers and of which we have already spoken in detail.

The number 13, beyond what was already said, permits us to go beyond the limiting patterns of time. The twenty-four-hour day, the sixty minutes, sixty seconds, and a year of twelve months, were created to confuse and limit us. Time can be bent, molded, stretched and contracted. We can sculpt each of our creations of time. As co-creators, the number 13 permits us to become masters of time through its holographic nature, freely creating life from infinite Loving that turns us, as humans, into the key that opens the door to access the highest vibration of light.

In addition to the previously said, the number 44, stands for loyalty. For us, that's loyalty to Light and firmness in our principles, not letting ourselves be confused, not giving power to exterior manipulation, namely fear. The number 44 is the unlimited belief in what we truly are: Love. It contains the power of Amen, which means to be firm, therefore it is the power of action, completely activated in the fifth mantra of IRB, which opens the second Nuclear Command.

The number 58, within the Hebrew table of the 72 names of God, corresponds to the *Shem Ha Mephorash*, which is also the name of Layer Thirteen. As Hurtak says in The 72 Sacred Names of God, this sacred name blesses and governs the human creation in all the inner mysteries of life and protects the evolution of the DNA, which is the ultimate goal of Layer Thirteen. Additionally, it is the combination of 5 and 8, which generates the movement of self-esteem, worthiness and empowerment of our true origins. It is constant evolution, endless movement, unlimited power.

4. Balance

It can be exhausting to sustain the totality of what we are without losing our balance. We are, after all, submitting ourselves to an experience of contradicting forces. Illness is a symptom of imbalance, and extremes unbalance us. Being balanced does not mean monotony or uniformity; it means to act and do from what we are, not reacting to what is happening in our exterior.

The day is a perfect complement to the night, the yin to the yang, allowing us to witness that when something is complete, balance manifests. To choose one or the other, to take part in the game of opposites, is to leave ourselves open to the feeling of being incomplete. Our balance is no longer harmonious, which can provoke a molecular breakdown in any of our parts.

I invite you to do this exercise: take a perfect sphere like a small ball of only one color and with no markings. Let us observe it for a few seconds. Now, with our eyes closed, let us rotate it in our mind's eye then look at it again. Would we be able to rotate it back to its original position? It is practically impossible to know which way we rotated the image. This doesn't happen so much because the sphere is symmetrical and uniform, but rather because it is very similar to what happens to our image in the mirror. If we were to swap places with our reflection in the mirror, no one would know the difference because our reflection is seemingly identical to our body. This type of symmetry or similarity reveals the sacred geometry that is the blueprint of the universe.

The universe as we know it, presents us with symmetry that controls the balance and stability of nature. A physical symmetry with which we are fairly familiar is the fact that electrical charges are both positive and negative. Like everything that surrounds us, we are composed of particles invisible to the naked eye that have positive and negative electric charges. The balance between these two charges permits us to live life without being electrocuted by our surroundings, which is composed of, among other things, electrical energy. This balance of opposing charges is what permits everything to flow and function in harmony within our universe.

We cannot say that all symmetry is "perfect," though the paradigmatic concept of IRB is that everything is perfect.

In art, the balance found in the masterpieces is carefully created by the great masters. And yet, not everything that has to do with balance has to do with exact symmetry; that is part of the change of paradigm. What we might call imperfection in some symmetries, is simply a characteristic of perfection in the properties of our universe. A human face, for example, as beautiful as it might be, can never be perfectly symmetrical; its beauty lies in the balance of its composition. This illustrates that the importance is not in similarity, but in the appropriate balance of creation.

Therefore, the balance proposed by IRB is not a symmetrical linear order; it is, on the contrary, to break the illusion of order, and to accept the world as is: completely unpredictable, where the origin and the result diverge. There is no one formula to fix the system because chaos is a part of order, and where the origin is, is the spark that generates creation.

Balance is the neutrality that embraces opposites to be complete, and only in completeness is there creation.

5. The Indigo Ray

According to Carroll and Tober (2001), who were the first people to introduce the concept of Indigo Children over twenty years ago, the Indigo vibration has simply been dormant for a long time. That is why IRB has come to awaken it. The number of Indigo Children has been steadily increasing for the last three or four generations, including the current one. The critical mass now vibrates completely in the Indigo frequency. Indigo Children are the confirmation of the future in the now; they are our present, and as adults we can tune into their purpose through IRB.

Many lightworkers don't even know that they have come here to sustain the Indigo frequency, yet many carry the Indigo or Violet-Indigo vibration. Their mission is to prepare the path and generate the understanding that this portal is now open. The Violet-Indigo ones form a bridge of understanding between the old and new vibrations, as they have a gift for working with both parts. Adults who have the Indigo frequency in their energetic fields have the characteristics of an Indigo child and must prepare the path; for me, particularly, as an Indigo adult my role has been to fully open a portal to new education, to relearn how certain things work on the physical plane: from the spiritual, from unlimited expression.

A great percentage of Indigo Children are considered a problem, especially in school, since the current educational system groups them together into diagnoses and demands they adjust to the norms. The individuality of these children is so strong that they reject any type of adjustment. What's important to them is to re-establish the group consciousness so as to activate its divine powers to create, change and form the new Earth. They are very special children, and their characteristics are sometimes difficult to manage for adults who do not open themselves to understanding the transparency and authenticity of Indigos. This is why it is important for adults to tune into the Indigo frequency and find balance in this vibration, instead of wanting to keep the children in a now-expired system of repression.

THIS IS THE TIME for us all to vibrate in the Indigo. The way that each of us experiences this frequency depends on the flexibility we have toward the new, and the openness with which we perceive the world. If we insist on remaining fixed in a philosophical, scientific, or religious structure, we may find that different aspects of our reality explode or implode completely and often suddenly. Many who have been distant or detached from these themes, may discover from one moment to the next an opening to new knowledge, infinite love for themselves and their surroundings, and a purpose in living which they have not understood before, that they haven't even suspected might exist on the other side of the veil. These are perhaps those who dare the most to connect to the Indigo essence. Indigo is synonymous with spontaneity and authenticity. Spontaneity does not follow the rules because it is an expression of consciousness, and consciousness is infinite Loving.

Therefore, the Indigo essence is the only one capable of transforming the programs of manipulation that have been written in our DNA and liberate it toward new states of consciousness and frequencies of ultra-high vibration.

The Indigo Ray allows us to detach and therefore free ourselves from the barriers of the norm, from the "I can't," from fears. It permits us to awaken from the hypnotic trance of the hologram that we have built, so that from consciousness we can build the hologram in which we want to continue to live, by completely remembering who we are in our true and infinite magnitude, and what we were created for. The subject of waking up from a hypnotic trance brings to mind the well-written trilogy "The Hunger Games, mentioned earlier when we talked about the hologram. IRB, with the power of the Indigo Ray, acts like a straight and unerring arrow, which at the end of Book Two the protagonist shoots into the air to break the frame of manipulation and war the twelve tribes have endured up to that point, giving birth to the thirteenth district.

The Indigo Ray activates our intuition, which knows how to make spontaneous decisions that lead to freedom, embracing everything while not identifying with anything. This is a unifying perspective, moving with the flow of knowledge. It's a way of being and knowing that language is incapable of expressing. It is to embrace all opposites so that from the center, from neutrality, we can simply love.

One night Roger, my partner on this path, in part, my soulmate and business partner, was reading something. We simultaneously channel this frequency, tune and information, and everything involving IRB. He was reading *Caballo de Troya* 9. Caná (Trojan

Horse 9. Cana, by J.J. Benítez, 2011). Suddenly he exclaimed, "Wait a minute! Stop! I want you to listen to this."

He began to read from a passage about a great healing miracle performed by Jesus, an event never before told by any of the evangelists, in which Jesus healed nearly 700 people that day, as described in great detailed by Benitez. A light blue metallic light broke through a heavy mass of clouds, and it was not a star. Everything became very still, and there was a great silence, then the waters of the lake rippled. An identical blue light appeared that seemed to be alive. After a deafening silence came over the crowd, a third ray appeared, this time white, striking the two previous ones. Then millions of points of blue light began to descend until absolutely everything was covered in blue: the streets, the houses, people, clothing, animals, hands, feet… It snowed blue!

The sensation experienced by those present was an overwhelming desire to cry (at this moment, you, dear reader, may be experiencing the same sensation). There were even tears that fell from the eyes of the Rabbi, as his disciples called Jesus. Then everything was covered in great darkness, and the natural sounds returned. This affected 683 people who in a matter of seconds were completely healed of all types of illness, from quadriplegia, to "incurable" genetic disorders, to "demon possession."

A few paragraphs later, Jesus is described as talking about the beauty and art of creation and about seeing the spirit behind the law, not the words, and he used a word for art that I loved the moment I heard it: bellinte, which means beauty and intelligence." That is what creation is, God's creation. Ours is a god that, according to Jesus, is a blue God that practices the religion of art: everything is the present because the future does not exist, and everything is devoted to Oneness, gifting light and immortality. Jesus then gave us a new concept of a kind, fatherly god and not a judgmental one.

When I heard this story, which for some may be fiction and for others a revision of the course of history, I found myself also covered in blue! Everything coincided with this information. Great healing is linked to the Blue Ray and infinite Compassion. Jesus performed healings when he tuned his will to the will of the creator, of the great artist, of Everything, from the place of purest Loving and infinite Compassion. Sound goes into profound reverence that manifests Presence. In its connection with Wisdom, a being simply tunes into the part of the ZPF where the hologram finds itself in perfect balance; there it activates its OMAK. Jesus is the greatest exponent of the OMAK on earth. My feeling while experiencing healings through the philosophy of IRB, has been an overwhelming desire to cry. I must confess, that is what I did when Roger finished reading the story.

6. Cordierite or "Iolite"

In those days of intense channeling, I found myself in Miami attending an international seminar. I enjoy assisting in these types of seminars, which serves to connect me to my superior essence. For me, these are moments of profound connection to the great universal intelligence from where everything is dictated.

Well, it was during one of those moments that I received the idea of the Bluewater Sapphire named "Iolite." As I said at the beginning of this book, I had the good fortune of training with Katrina Raphaell in the art of crystals, so I considered myself knowledgeable on the matter; yet, the name and essence of the crystal being shown to me at that moment were completely unknown. I shared this information with Roger, who was still reading the *Cana* saga; at that precise moment he was on the pages that described the scene when the master reunited all his disciples and asked them to kneel, and when he raised his eyes and arms to the blue sky, everything was silent. All that could be heard was his great voice consecrating his disciples and himself to the will of Ab-ba (what Jesus called his father). When the master finished the prayer of consecration, he placed in the left hand of each of his disciples a blue stone, and Iolite, and at that precise moment a flock of pelicans flew over them. For them pelicans represented total and authentic Love.

For me this was a great confirmation. Everything I have written in this book is the result of years of surrender and acceptance of my mission and that the Universe, God, the Being, Presence, Source, or however we might word it, was confirmed through this message of synchronicity and the power that IRB brings to the planet, recovering the true teachings that were distorted by religion through the years but are revealed once more from the vision of new and unlimited power to convert Love into a reality.

However, despite this momentous experience that I was going through, my curiosity did not find a different option from corroborating the information through someone who I believed knew a lot about crystals; actually, it was the person who has always provided me with the most beautiful crystals in my collection: Ernesto Pereira, Uruguayan-born and Colombian raised. Ernesto is a dear friend of mine, someone who walks the path beside me. So I e-mailed him asking about Iolite. He responded a few minutes later, describing its characteristics, plus promising to have one for me when I returned to Bogotá.

What I learned about Iolite is that it is a precious stone of blue tones that evoke a profound indigo, some with a little white and others leaning more toward gray. They say the Vikings used Iolite as a polarizer to locate the sun on cloudy days, aiding navigation on the high seas. I find that metaphor to be beautiful, for Iolite also shows us the light in the middle of darkness. In ancient times it was known as "water sapphire," a term no longer used, though that is how it was revealed to me. In *The Crystal Bible* (Hall, 2007), I found the following information:

> Iolite is a vision stone. It activates the third eye and facilitates visualization and intuitive insight when all the chakras are in alignment. It is used in shamanic ceremonies and aids journeys out of the body. In contact with the auric field, Iolite gives off an electrical charge that re-energizes the field and aligns with the subtle bodies. It helps to understand and let go of the reasons for addiction, and to express the true I. Purifies thoughts. It helps to alleviate discord in relationships, as it motivates us to take responsibility for ourselves, also helping us to overcome codependence in relationships. Used in healing, it creates a strong constitution, reduces deposits of fat in the body, relieves the effects of alcohol and aids the detoxification and regeneration of the liver. This stone treats malaria, fevers, sinus congestion and breathing problems, as it helps to eliminate bacteria and alleviate migraines[…]

After reading this transcript, I understood why Iolite had been given to me as part of IRB, and I could not wait to see Ernesto so I could receive one, feel it, work with it and connect to the information it had for me. After arriving in Bogotá, my first visit was to see my Uruguayan friend who had a box of Iolites for me, marked: Cordierite. At that moment, it was as if the box and I had a déjà vu moment going back to the time of the Master Jesus and that moment written of by J.J. Benitez. At once information that came to me, a phrase repeated many times by the priest at my childhood church: "I am the Lamb of God who takes away the sin of the world. Blessed are those called to this dinner. I am not worthy to receive you in my house, but one word from you and all shall be healed." At that moment, everything in the little gem store became blue for me. Tears fell from my eyes, and in that moment I had no more questions, only understanding.

The Cordierite, as I like to call her, is a great companion; she requires no sacrifice, nor killing a lamb so that the sins of the world may be healed (since there are no sins but only decisions that allow us to experience from our own creation), and she is there to share in the banquet, the celebration, the oneness, to "free" us from karma in a new concept of pure creation from Loving. She is there as a reminder, to amplify the light when we find ourselves in the darkness, to remind us that the creator within us is blue, is art, is bellinte. This is why she is a fundamental part of the initiation in IRB.

Fabiana Londoño, my great friend and a follower of IRB since its beginnings, handmade a beautiful bracelet of cordierites that I always wear now. It is my way of remembering the Indigo light that illuminates everything and the Master Jesus when he initiated his disciples.

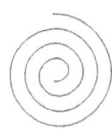

Chapter XXII
The Four Pillars of Activation

There are not many paths. There are many names to the same path, and that path is Consciousness.

Osho

1. Love

There are different possible attitudes toward love; you can eat it, drink it, breathe it, but you can also live it. Those that eat it stay within the physical plane and never find satisfaction, as they're settling for lower pleasures. The pleasure of those who drink love is less raw, but they're still confined to the delights and satisfactions of a lower (the astral) plane. Those who breathe love are philosophers, writers and artists, who have reached the mental plane; love is their constant source of inspiration. Only those who live love, in the subtle and ethereal dimensions of love, truly possess it. For them love is the light of the mind and the heat of the heart, and they spread light and warmth over all those around them. Those who live in this love, live in plenitude.

Omraam Mikhaël Aïvanhov

When there is no difference between you and me, when we float in absolute Unity, we experience integration, and that is how we understand infinite Love. From love's essence, we have the power to transcend without losing ourselves. This is not the same as loving from feeling; infinite loving goes beyond anything imaginable;

it doesn't form roots because it identifies itself with the root, the sprout, the stem, the blossom, in the All, in Everything. It does not need to possess, for being One with Everything, nothing belongs to it. Infinite Love is simply a part of that Everything, or of nothing. It does not suffer because it only accepts and surrenders to the purest essence of each moment. It does not generate attachments, or discriminates; it is not selective; infinite Love transcends genders, species, dimensions, distances and time. That Love we are talking about lives, is, and manifests at all times with everyone and everything that surrounds it, without exception, starting with ourselves. Love is not an emotion; it is an energy.

When one lives and breathes the energy of Love, nothing any longer matters, nothing is sought; everything is. We live in the here and now, knowing that the only permanent thing is evolution, manifesting, creation, infinity, and we choose that which we call joy long before we experience it because it is in the Field. We have simply chosen it to live in the eternal present, from total consciousness. It is the engine that permits us to transcend paradigms, with the clear understanding that mistakes do not exist, only opportunities to learn, whether voluntary or not; we must simply know how to create everything from the heart.

Loving, in its true context, is balance itself, a balance of Everything, of what is and is not, the part and the whole; it is Oneness, Wisdom and Compassion, Presence and Consciousness; it is a manifestation of all possibilities, it is synchronicity, it is perfection. Loving is enthusiasm, it is spontaneity, and the spontaneity of the music of Spirit; Love is inspiration of unity, of detachment; it is the silence between thoughts. It's the pure silence of Consciousness, and Consciousness does not need to think, as it simply knows.

Love harmonizes our DNA beyond the worlds of illusion and sings along with the superior resonances of major octaves, vibrating at the highest frequencies. Love harmonizes us with truth and thereby frees us, permitting us to access new levels of consciousness, of infinite Consciousness that facilitates the total activation of our DNA. This maintains the vibration of freedom, health, and abundance that can only lead to joy. Love is the only laser that allows us to see "reality" in a different way.

> TO LOVE ONESELF IS THE BEGINNING OF A LIFELONG ROMANCE.
> Oscar Wilde

Love yourself! Love what you create from who you are! Love the evolution that turned you into who you are each moment! When you love, you are loved; when this happens, you are Love!

2. Presence

Beyond the thousand-and-one ways that life manifests in this dimension, constantly appearing and disappearing, there exists an emptiness where everything is creative potential. Creation is Consciousness manifesting as life, never to be erased. It is not born, nor does it die; it is infinite and is always present. Throughout this book we have talked about the word of God and the power it contains, as witnessed by many religions, norms, laws and conditions. We have also understood, as we reach these later pages, that we are part of that which we call God, and that it is pretty much what we are, no matter the name we want to give it. We can call it Essence, Self, Life, Consciousness, Infinite, or Emptiness. Further, everything we see as manifest creation is the infinite occupying the finite; it is that spirit that encloses the physical, the essence of all forms that fill, visibly or invisibly, what we call emptiness.

The existence of everything lies in its being. Presence is the consciousness of being, of untainted permanence. It is only by being present in the here, in the now, that we can tune into that state, using that part of the field that contains the information about who we are. Silence is the vehicle that permits us to listen to the quietness of being, of being as the experience itself that elevates us to pleasure and into a state of permanent joy. The self that is consciousness never understands through the mind because we're talking about a direct experience, unique and distinctive. The main obstacle to experiencing this unity, this connection to the being, with Presence, is the mind, which ceaselessly generates emotions, images, beliefs and perceptions. The mental noise that keeps us from finding the state of stillness and silence necessary to the experience of Presence, which is nothing more than being present.

This is why Presence is a fundamental part of IRB, which does not propose that we live as hermits to be able to experience the Four Pillars, but simply to live everyday life in pure consciousness in each moment.

To live in Presence permits us to consciously recognize each event, without the veil of illusion of time or ego, the aim being to permanently experience consciousness in the present moment, in constant connection with the power of the inner Presence. Only Presence permits us to go on the sacred path that leads us to consciously activating the power of being who we truly are, to remain tuned into the part of the ZPF where we create with unlimited potential, from a new perception of reality, for the common creation of the new Earth.

To remain conscious of the present moment is a state of being, not a state of doing. In this way Presence permits us to experience any type of moment with gratitude borne of consciousness of acceptance. There is no attachment or rejection but only gratitude and integration, because all is Love. Being conscious of the present moment is not an idea that the mind creates, not yet another thought, but a form of living in itself, in experience, in attitude, a way of being that does not imply any type of effort but, on the contrary, permits us to respond to situations from the totality of our being, of what we truly and freely are. Presence is the perfect door to accessing Totality.

3. Compassion

Compassion is, above all, the path that connects us to the All. When we are in a state of compassion, we do not feel separate. Compassion allows the activation of the Unity and creation for the All. Compassion is intimately linked to acceptance, and acceptance is made up of patience; they cannot exist separately, as nothing does.

True compassion has nothing to do with what we often call pity. It is not about sympathizing with someone who is suffering. In reality, compassion means taking the necessary action steps to help. We can give the proper example or encourage others to establish the supreme state of being in which we can stop being victims to the desire for suffering and tune into complete joy. Teaching does not mean coming up with an entire repertory of words and rhetoric for each moment of the day; rather it means to provide an example and demonstrate coherence, not only with our physical eyes but also beyond the senses, openly, so as to be able to speak from the heart. We radiate the love that comes from Compassion, permitting us to respect the dignity of the human being in front of the greatness of the unlimited universe of life. Compassion applies being able to teach freedom from duality over illusion; it is unlimited, which is why it coexists with the Infinite.

This also does not imply getting involved with trying to change the other person's process, but to be a pure instrument of service, available when and as needed. In the old energy it was believed that the work of a spiritual master was to give up to his or her last drop of blood and sweat so that others would be conscious of their lives. This has activated programs in the DNA such as: "Everything related to spirituality must be free;" "The master belongs to his disciples;" "Lightworkers should not charge fees;" and "Money does not go along with a spiritual life;" which misconceptions have made it so that people with great developed gifts — which we all have — work hard at jobs they do not love, just so they can survive, leaving very little time to the growth and recognition of the light in our being, wasting our linear time instead of doing what we should truly be doing. This constitutes a program of manipulation, which completely takes us out of IRB.

Compassion begins with ourselves. When we realize we have an array of tools and enough consciousness to walk our own path, we begin to be the instrument of life that gives the example and the framework for others to follow, into a new vibration of deserving, where suffering is no longer an option in life.

To simply feel sorry, or even to cry for others, is not Compassion. Many times this might actually be an act of pride. For it to be true Compassion, it is necessary to know that we all possess an infinite Wisdom for connecting to the supreme essence, as vehicles to the paradise we each deserve. To empathize with someone is to give that person something they are not able to give themselves at that time, so that they never have to depend on anyone for it again. It's like the saying: "Give a man a fish and he will eat for a day; teach a man to fish and he will eat for a lifetime." This requires taking into account all existences, all manifestations of life equally and permitting all, including those whom we believe to have no sensibility (due to not being human) to awake within themselves the magic of sharing.

When Master Jesus healed others, he did so through the Compassion he felt for the leper, the blind and the dying. It was not pity. The Compassion experienced by this extraordinary being elevated the frequency of the person seeking healing to the frequency of the Father, where their absolute perfection was recognized, and the patient found him or herself perfectly healed. That is how we recognize our own divine essence, from our true origin, and help others recognize themselves in the same way, remaining in a state of perfection.

The human being is an integration of systems. In this dimension, for example, we are a system within another, such as the family system, the neighborhood system, the city, province or state, and so on — all of them composed of systems such as the physical, the emotional, the mental and the spiritual. There are, of course, many others that we won't go into in detail. In other words, we are a microcosms in the macro–cosms, and the macro-cosms of our inner micro-cosms. When something changes in one of the systems, because we are connected, one way or another every system is affected. The movie The Butterfly Effect (2004, written and directed by Eric Bress) illustrates the idea that any type of change can cause a very large wave.

When we activate Compassion in the totality of our systems, we use the necessary frequency or vibration and the necessary language. Since we are all One, diversity speaks in many languages, which instead of separating us, completes us. That is why IRB speaks in the language of the heart; it is the only universal language, and Love is the best vehicle for its comprehension. In the mass healing scene orchestrated by Master Jesus in Benitez's Cana, we understand that it was the biggest act of Compassion ever carried out, capable of transforming realities without words, without anything external, through a strong and pure connection with the supreme being of each person, or the origin of its OMAK. That is activated at a hundred percent. Compassion does not require words, but supreme acts.

The most effective form of support that we can offer to elevate any human being from absolute Compassion to a plane where healing exists in all its aspects, is to be that vehicle in touch with the supreme part of each person, both at an individual and group level, so that the activated being uses their powers of guidance based on their precise evolutional moment and purpose, igniting the light forever. This is the greatest act of Compassion that can be manifest in daily life for the good of all beings.

The purer, clearer and firmer the contact with the highest essence of each person where we are all One in Living Light and Loving, the more supreme and complete becomes the vehicle of Compassion, which ignites the light that illuminates the density that has kept so many beings immersed in suffering, where lack is a part of reality.

> Unified action is to completely communicate with the world in which we are living. Each moment is new, full and complete. Each element of this world deserves respect. A pine grows on a rock. Invisible drops of dew give life to a desert. There is no separation, no concept of big or small, no anxious searching, no fear. Unified action is to forget the self and "allow the Ganges' sands to run through our fingers." To be in unity with the people who practice the way, and with those who do not practice it, is to be in unity with whatever we find, without duality.
>
> Buddhist Principle

4. Wisdom

Wisdom is how we set the mind aside and leave a space for intuition. Our true reality is in Presence rather than misinterpretations. Our intuition develops as Wisdom toward everything that is, to its actual totality. It is seeing and knowing, free of expectations. When we awaken this facility, we are free: free of concepts, free of limits, free of dense beliefs, free of separation and of guilt — free to create from the greatness of who we are, not from the control that we believe we have. We are part of a universe that totality controls, not in a universe that controls totality.

Wisdom has nothing to do with knowledge. Knowledge is a series of concepts stored in the mind. Wisdom, on the other hand, is action, is creation. Wisdom frees and illuminates the mind; it is pleasure; it is open, clear and unlimited, never born nor does it die. Wisdom is timeless and unconditional; it bestows totality. When the teaching of the mirror of the mind is incorporated, Wisdom remains within us in a lasting manner, as it ceases to oscillate between joy and suffering conditioned by pleasure and displeasure, as it understands the depths that exist behind both. Wisdom understands that the All is free, free of rigid pre-established concepts, free of false beliefs, and free of the shadow of lived experiences.

Wisdom is attained by tuning in beyond our thoughts. Its timeless essence, consciousness, resides right in that empty space found between thoughts, behind thoughts. Wisdom knows thoughts. When we become aware of that space through Presence, we recognize all the external and internal as freely available, and that is where we experience Truth and find wisdom.

Wisdom is comprehension itself, beyond ego; it is the first thing that emerges in the state of radiant consciousness that cannot be perturbed by anything or anyone. Wisdom simply happens. It is the enlightened acceptance of the non-reality of everything external, it is non-duality, the self-complete information that lives in the "emptiness;" it is flow. It is constant and infinite change.

It is also absolute comprehension that the subject, the object, and the event, are all aspects of the same totality and are infinitely interconnected, generating mutual growth and learning. It is the understanding of the perfection of everything; it is to not judge, not to criticize, not to want change, but just flow in an endless dance of events in the sweet transformation of what Is. Wisdom is imperturbability; it is peace. It is permitting thoughts, emotions, actions, and words that follow this state to transform reactive habits. Wisdom knows that habits end up wanting to control and to perpetuate suffering and attachment, which in the end are the same thing.

Suffering is the difference between our expectations and what actually happens. To expect things is to jump ahead of the event, not to live in the present, filling the mind with predictive thoughts that take us out of tune with the present, thus blocking us from the wisdom needed to live in the present. While attachment is to want everything to remain the same unconditionally, as though it belonged to us, and attempting to block evolution, change and transformation, and to witness the impossibility that this is to see our suffering as what it is.

Wisdom is knowing that we have the power to access the necessary information at the right time, without trying to accumulate knowledge, because it is always available in the moment. To want to be attached to that information is to deny the possibility of evolution and so it becomes just knowledge, far from being Wisdom. The latter allows us to remain in tune with the part of the ZPF where there are no veils, filters or obstacles to misrepresent reality.

Wisdom is the container of everything; it lives in everything and is the mother of creation, turning neutral space into the most exciting of realities.

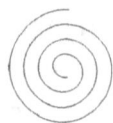

Chapter XXIII
Transcending Paradigms

Past and future obviously have no reality of their own. Just as the moon has no light of its own but can only reflect the light of the sun, so past and future are only pale reflections of the light, power and reality of the eternal present. Their reality is "borrowed" from the Now.

Eckhart Tolle

1. Stop Humanizing God's Image

There has been a vast mythology created around God, and it has been firmly anchored all over the planet. It is everywhere, in every dogma and religion, regardless of how they differ from each other. How can we imagine God, the creative source of the universe? How can we imagine a power that is in every being, in each breath of life? How can we imagine something that has neither beginning nor end? How do we describe the entire universe in a tiny fraction of time? How do we imagine a Father God who exists in the totality, in the eternal, manifested in each particle of every being?

Humanity has been taught that God possesses human attributes; therefore, God has feelings: He punishes, rewards, gets angry, feels offended, likes or dislikes this or that….

Quantum physics does not argue with itself; it has mapped out a very congruent system, and its approach to unity cannot be denied. The energy that for eons we have called god is only energy without polarization because it is the singularity from which everything is created. When we are born on this planet, we learn all kinds of limiting concepts meant to keep us separated from God's energy since they teach that we must permanently work on ourselves in order to get closer to God, as if He were a separate entity far removed from us. It is at that moment that we draw the veil of forgetfulness and separate ourselves from the essence that has no duality, only Love. We are God. We are Love. To say that we must "get closer to God" is to imply that God is far from us, and separate. It is to deny our divine indivisible essence. We are part of the All; therefore, we are a manifestation of God, whatever name or label we wish to give God. We are going to talk about God because that is the title of the paradigm.

The old paradigm mandates that we must behave this or that way to become acceptable to Divinity, and the majority of the dogmas instill belief in suffering, sacrifice, isolation, poverty, sickness, and vows that supposedly lead to Paradise. All of these dogmas agree on one thing: human beings were created in God's image. That belief misleads many to think that God possesses human qualities, instead of understanding that humans can possess Godlike qualities by recognizing our divine nature. As taught by the old paradigm, we have humanized God, attaching human characteristics to God's image.

How does the old paradigm depict beings of light such as angels? We have given them human faces, skin color, wings, and even names. The old paradigm labels everything so the logical mind can comprehend it. That in itself is also part of the paradigm. In consciousness, there are only energies that form part of the totality and whose mission is to make themselves manifest through channels that interpret their messages. We give them names so that we can relate to them. Those energies may be the channels' highest essence bringing a message of evolution through their own higher selves. Kryon, for instance, in a channeling through Lee Carroll, explained that "Kryon" is a collective energy from the other side of the veil, given a name so that humanity can relate to it; however, it may be a different energy every time. As the channels clear their filters, the purity of God changes accordingly in the messages.

Within the totality, there are no individual entities. There are energies, including angelic energies. Some we have named Michael, Gabriel, Uriel, Rafael, and so on, to whom we have projected qualities such as power, masculinity, healing, wings, swords, flames, and colors like blue, white, gold or green. We have done this so that we can better relate to the infinite. All archangels known to us are part of the All, and just as perfect as the All. Anytime one of them "speaks," he does so on behalf of all the angelic energies, who offer very similar messages about Love. Angels are never in conflict among themselves. They only want to show us specific attributes that exist within each of us, attributes that lay dormant most of the time. When we recognize these attributes in the angels, we can activate them within ourselves.

Angelic entities are never in conflict with each other, or with the masters, or with the light essence, because they form part of the Heavenly host, just as you and I do. Nothing is separate. Nothing exists independently. Those of us who have incarnated as humans have manifested through a physical body, and we may have names that differentiate us from others, though of course we are unique in the highest essence of our being. We are all One with the Living Light and Love. All messages come from the same source where we Are All One. The message resonates in our physical body because the divine part of the human being is part of the All, and as we receive a truthful message, we simultaneously radiate it and share it. Only when we are clear of filters, veils, obstacles and limitations, can we resonate with the message. IRB helps with the elimination of these filters and veils, to achieve a pure and clear connection with the highest essence of our being, where we are One in the Living Light and Love, to connect with that part of the ZPF where all the infinite potentials are available to everyone.

The belief in conflict is part of the old paradigm. We have warred with one another to defend religious beliefs; we have even fought "holy wars." THIS IS THE TIME to learn that there is no polarity in God. There are no fallen angels. All the stories are part of an old paradigm and the old energy that became part of humanity. They were tools to help us understand the light and the darkness, which are not two separate things. There is no division in Light. Love is pure; it is the source of all creation; therefore, there is no conflict. All the myths and legends were created as a source of understanding or as a source of manipulation. When we fill our "logical" minds with preconceived ideas, we deny ourselves the capacity to feel, to connect with the Oneness, with the Infinite Source of the heart, the only capacity that can keep us connected with the information of the cosmos.

To transcend the old paradigm means to accept that we are part of an indivisible, perfect, majestic, splendid, non-divided and non-polarized Oneness. The fight against the devil, evil and darkness, is over. There is duality in the human physicality only because of our beliefs; this duality was implanted in the old grid with which we created the Earth. With the new Christic energy that descends through IRB, we discover the pure and divine Love of God, a love that has never been polarized.

THIS IS THE TIME to stop humanizing God and to begin divinizing the human. Only by transcending the old paradigms, the old beliefs, the old energy and the old manipulative myths, are we able to access the information from the Totality and live in Love, Presence, Compassion and Wisdom.

2. The Meaning of Responsibility

Responsibility is something very different from the concept we learned in the old paradigm. We can continue to call it responsibility while gaining a different understanding of its meaning and practical application in the present moment. Responsibility is not what we practiced in the old energy. What we did was carry the weight of adulthood, carry others' guilt and our own, punish and sabotage ourselves for everything we thought we had to do but couldn't or didn't want to do, including cleansing ourselves of "sins" we never even committed. To be responsible in the new energy is to understand the results we generate with each of our thoughts, words, emotions and actions. When we understand this, we stop being victims of circumstances and can create change if we are not satisfied with the results.

Without a doubt, we are responsible for the whole spectrum of who we are. Whether something "good" or "bad" happens, we are responsible for it. In the old paradigm, we were taught that "if something bad happened, it was our fault. If something good happened, it was God's will." I invite you, dear reader, to stop reading for a moment and take a trip down memory lane. Think about everything you have consciously achieved until now; everything you were able to do, everything that brought disharmony to your life yet you were able to transform. Think about the times you were sick or felt discomfort, and you were able to get well. Think of the experiences that you thought painful at the time, but later you knew were the best thing that could have happened. Think about this: if that had not happened, how would your life be now? Reflect on these bridges that, even though they caused you initial problems, you were strong enough to cross. Think about the times when temptation was very strong, yet you maintained your integrity. Now the question is, "Who did all that?" Ask yourself, "Was it me?" The answer is, "Yes!" This is the time to acknowledge that. "I did it! And I was able to do it because divine power is in me."

We have in ourselves the power to rewrite the attributes of our personality, to transform anything that has happened, to incorporate the lesson into our DNA and change our perspective, And to recover the consciousness of past lives, the information of future or parallel lives, allowing our present consciousness to resolve anything that comes up. To face your strength, all your natural gifts, and everything you thought you did not have. Once we understand that all the information is part of the All and that we are the All, everything is possible here and now.

THIS IS THE TIME to accept responsibility. We must be responsible for all the good things in our lives, and even for those things we perceived as bad, because in the new paradigm, after you receive IRB in your life, the creation of our world will be entirely our responsibility — without veil, filters or interference.

In the old energy, we even criticized our own consciousness. How many times have we thought that something far off was our responsibility? That, if a change was required, it had to begin with us and no one else? THIS IS THE TIME to stop and see what we have done to ourselves, to take responsibility for everything we have created. This is the time to celebrate our creations and congratulate ourselves because we deserve it. The moment has come to change what does not provide comfort, because we deserve the best. THIS IS THE TIME to become both divine and responsible.

3. Creating from the Present

As we stated early in this book, fear is a hypothesis that refers to the future. Anytime we think of the future, we do so in the present, which is the only reality that exists. So, then, let us chose in the present what we want to happen in the future. Let us rewrite the drama of the past, which is stored in our cells and is generating an energy that could potentially cause us to repeat the past. If the present that we lived in the past was not pleasant, does it make sense to keep bringing it to the present if we don't want it in the future? The present could actually be the future that has come back, or the past nothing more than the present lived in another moment, taking information from another time.

THIS IS THE TIME to change the information in our cells; we do not erase it because we would be forsaking what we have learned. Let us observe the past with the wisdom we've gained as masters and understand that we do not have to continue learning from those same experiences. Let us create some new ones. We do not have to erase or reprogram anything; we only have to create what we want by bringing the information from IRB into our cells now. When we fear the future because we think this or that will happen, our thoughts are writing the future. However, if we are overcome by fear because of what we sense will happen in the future, and we are unable to change the potential of our thoughts, we can then access this future before it occurs and modify it. We cannot access this new perception operating from fear; it must be accessed from the creative self.

Fear paralyzes everything that, as divine beings and protagonists in our own play, we came to fulfill. This is really a lack of responsibility. Let us shatter, then, the paradigm of fear and write each present moment of our life within the energy of Love. Let us be born anew each second. Each moment is an opportunity to create a magical experience. Do not let fear stop you but rather empower it with Love and Living Light. Part of our responsibility within the new paradigm is to see God in everything. If God is in everything, then each of us is God. As Lee Carroll writes in the Book II of Kryon, "Don't think like a human anymore."

We invest more energy rejecting what we do not want to happen, than focusing on creating what our Universal Will came here to fulfill.

Once we understand that we can create anything in alignment with our Divinity, it is imperative to leave behind the concept of linear time that freezes us in the past or make us fear the future. That almost implies that we must learn to write, think and speak differently since everything is in the present. When we say, "it was" or "it will be," neither is true. It always "is," the moment something happens, always in the present. When we live in the "is," we harmonize with our own eternity.

We have the power to modify our future and the future of our planet if we create a different collective potential together. We are experiencing an endless number of extremely dangerous collective potentials. If we avoid our co-creative responsibility, we bring such disasters closer without even knowing it. Living consciously with, and believing in, the supreme essence of our being and operating in alignment with it, enables the greatest light potentials for our lives, enlightening those around us. Learning to receive messages from our supreme essence and trusting them is an essential part of this new information. When we modify the grid of our supreme essence, we modify the framework that interconnects us with everything that is part of our world. When we assume responsibility to co-create from consciousness, we co-create for the totality.

To listen properly to the instructions from our supreme essence, it is necessary to quieten the noises in our head, to be in a state of peace, on center, and receive them with our hearts. Many times these messages manifest in our dreams. Even though we are not always conscious of them, the next day when we are awake, we may know exactly the right way to co-create what we want.

We do not always have to wait until we fall asleep to receive messages from our dreams. The meditations, music and mantras of IRB help us achieve the same effect, tuning us (after the initiation that teaches these principles) into that essence, a connection that allows us to easily observe the new reality when we accept responsibility for being the creators of our manifestations. Nevertheless, a vital part of your success lies in letting go of control over the results, in the same way that you don't even think about walking, eating, breathing or perspiring. Simply allow the future to continuously actualize the potentials of the present in Presence and Consciousness. What this means is that we must generate a consciousness wherein our past, present and future, are three simultaneous realities happening at different speeds.

From the present, we can change the way we view the past. In the same way, we can bring information from the future to create the present. In other words, the present is the Zero Point Field where all the information generated by the infinite mirror converges, and when we access the ZPF, we create without limits, just as in the reflection of a pair of mirrors (an infinity mirror) set up in a recursive manner.

The secret lies at the central point where everything resides in the purest and most loving coexistence. At that center, in that present, we find Layer Thirteen of the DNA conducting the orchestra of all the realities that converge in our being and setting and actualizing in the present any potential future. It is also the composer of our past, hence the importance of being responsible in the resonance of a high vibrational frequency. Without a conductor to keep the orchestra in tune with the consciousness of Love, Presence, Compassion and Wisdom, our cellular system plays a solitary tune, returning to chaos and separation.

Let us go even farther. It is important that, when we create from the ZPF — Layer Thirteen of our DNA, the quantum conductor

— we apply that same sense of responsibility, and what we create for ourselves, we also create for the collective. When we create potentials for the collective that oppose ours, again we are responsible for planetary chaos. We are competitive beings, and as long as there is competition there will be disorder. Instead let us join in cooperation. If we do not take care of the planetary balance, we will again fall prey to the ego, and since our bodies react before the planet, we will again tune into the energy of illness, which is a reflection of imbalance. Remember the axiom, "Our own perception of time and space is just an illusion."

4. Changing Traditions

We must stop focusing on everything that operates under the old energy, under the limits, the fears, the impositions and the rules that once forced us to believe in something untrue, or to do something against our will. We must stop thinking about those untruths, and speaking of them, and even feeling them.

When we are infants, we depend on someone to feed, dress, bathe and take us places. When we grow up, we can do those things for ourselves, and in our own personal way, yet we tend to hold onto that feeling of love and care given to us in the past. We stay with the things that resonate with our own style and change the things that don't. During our adolescence, we rebel against everything. We want to listen to our own music, dress in our own style, do our hair the way we like it, perhaps with a color different from anyone else's in the family. It means that when we grow up and connect with our essence, we live our lives in accordance with our own criterion. Unfortunately, there are those who still live by someone else's rules. Only those who dare to be different, who dare to change their own paradigm, will achieve connection and evolution.

I ask you, dear reader, would you, at this moment and your present age, play the same games you played as a child? Would you study the same algebra book you had in the ninth grade? Would it make sense? If you already learned them, there is no point in going over the same lessons, correct? What, then, is your present reality?

THIS IS THE TIME to establish a new common sense, at the age you are now, escaping the senseless traditions that trapped us in the past. The energy has changed, the old ceremonies and rituals, as fun as they might still be, are no longer necessary. We must travel very light now, without anchors, without paradigms, without ties, so that we can always live in the present, filled with ancestral wisdom. Let us begin to remember the future so that we can manifest it in the present.

We are creating a new Earth, and we are bold pioneers, but this time we do it without wars and abuse. We are as wise indigenous and aboriginal peoples creating a new beginning in a new energy. IRB supplies the necessary tools for us to be protagonists in a new beginning of 26,000 years of history. To achieve this, it is necessary to change the traditions, to rewrite them or, better yet, abolish them. When we keep doing the same things because of tradition, we continue trimming the ham without knowing why. It is necessary to become mature without losing the authenticity of the child. Let us become responsible with the freshness of the new. Traditions are for humans. Divinity does not institute traditions.

5. Nothing to Protect Ourselves from

Did you know that to produce light, a conventional light bulb must have an electrical current that switches on-and-off every half second? Even though we think the light is continuous, it is formed by alternating light and darkness. The old paradigms have us believing that darkness is sinister and that we must protect ourselves from this dark energy. The concept is so deeply imbedded that it lives even in those who have dedicated their lives to healing and to support those who want to regain their vitality through light and Love. Many healers speak of protection to avoid entanglement with the dark energies patients may bring with them; their fear of catching a spiritual disease drives them to perform a series of "protection" rituals.

The abyss of forgetfulness is so deep that it prevents us from seeing the true reality. Have we ever seen the sun worried about finding shelter because night is approaching? Have you not realized that as soon as the sun rises, darkness fades? Have you not noticed all the things you have to do to darken a room in the middle of the day? We close doors and shutters, we cover cracks… yet, if there is even a tiny hole that lets the light in, there can be no darkness. All you have to do is turn on a lamp or light bulb or light a candle, and everything is visible again.

Fear has been instilled to separate us from our true divine nature. Love illuminates everything in its path. When we think, speak, feel and act with Love, we do not have to fight against anything because we accept the darkness as part of reality and we learn to give light continually, allowing the same darkness to become a generator of light, as does a light bulb. There is no struggle; there is only flow, acceptance and love. A candle does not protect itself but only transforms darkness into light. Let us be light by keeping ourselves in the highest vibrations of the Living Light, so that the light never goes out. If light is alive and eternal, it shines forever.

On the other hand, thanks to the darkness of night, we can gaze at the stars. Thus, there are things we can only see with the light, but there other spectacular lights that only shine brightly in the dark. There are different degrees of dimness and brightness for each situation. Only totality is perfection, and perfection is not comparable to protection.

6. Seeing Things Differently

At the time of Copernicus, people believed that the sun revolved around the Earth. Finally it was demonstrated that the sun is a star almost a hundred million miles from Earth. Actually it was the Earth, along with the other planets, that revolved around this local star. Despite knowing this, we still say that the sun rises in the east and sets in the west, as if we still held the old belief that the sun revolves around us.

We rush to watch the sunset, but we are not really aware that the sun is not "going down;" we ourselves are moving away until we can no longer see it. Every day we wait for the sun to rise so that we can get up and begin our daily labors. How would our reality change if we felt the constant movement that creates the illusion that we see or don't see the sun? Well, that is one of the many realities happening in our daily lives hidden by the old paradigms or simply by the way we continue perceiving it. The truth is not that the sun comes out and then hides. It seems that our reality is the same because we haven't changed the way we perceive or describe the sunset. Although that does not seem very relevant, our entire reality can change a great deal if we perceive it from another point of view. We then become participants in a totally different reality or truth. THIS IS THE TIME to accept that only by setting aside our limited points of view and allowing ourselves to go into space, can we see that the sun neither comes out nor goes away but shines perpetually.

A part of ourselves sees everything from a higher point of view, like a traffic helicopter or a radio broadcast indicating which routes are open or jammed, helping motorists avoid traffic jams, accidents and interruptions. When we walk linearly within our beliefs system, always taking the same road we have traveled before, without listening to the guides who have a road map, we can lose our way or unnecessarily get stuck in delays. THIS IS THE

TIME to become aware of our higher being and operate from there, to tune into the ZPF, within which exists the potential of the light we are trying to manifest.

It is very simple; everything we truly want to manifest is possible within the boundless possibilities available to us. To achieve this, it is necessary to see the familiar with new eyes. We cannot change events, but we can change the way we see and handle them. We can also rewrite our histories when we perceive them differently from this moment. Let us change our perspectives and broaden our vision; let us take a step back and contemplate the totality. We can stop being puppets in the hands of those who want to manipulate our divinity. Only when we are connected to the All, can we create without limits.

When we remain in sacred consciousness, working from the totality of who we are, from the most supreme part our being where we are all one with Love and the Living Light, we never risk taking the wrong road, much less misleading anyone, because we are always assured of the best present moment, each instant. We have the full assurance and confidence that everything is happening in keeping with our ultimate creation, for the highest good. We do not label anything as positive or negative since we accept that everything that happens is absolutely perfect. Perfection is another paradigm we can change when our view changes. When we judge perfection from our old preconceived belief system, there is labeling of good and bad, beautiful and ugly, and an endless list of other polarities.

In the Oneness, everything is perfect, even that which we may have judged as harmful. In our next moment, we understand that it is part of a process toward a more perfect outcome. When we are in tune with the highest essence of our being, the resonance is always for the highest good, regardless of the package in which it arrives. IRB allows us to stay in complete balance with this harmony and remember that we can create changes arising from the structure of something, but not from the change in it but because the object is basically timeless.

> THINGS ARE AS THEY ARE, THEY ARE NOT WHAT WE THINK ABOUT THEM
> Zen Principle

7. There is Nothing to Heal

Within the perfection of what we are, our true origin, there is nothing to heal. We are healthy, we are perfect, and we have access to all information. We need only to open our consciousness to this knowledge through IRB, and activate that spacecraft that allows us to move through our multidimensionality and find the right place for each state of consciousness at the required moment. This is perhaps the biggest paradigm that must be changed in order to connect to the divine perfection of who we really are and begin to enjoy the OMAK and the ZPF.

And so it is!

LOVE IS BLUE

Epilogue

Everything written in this book is intended for you to feel. Utilize the language as a key to open the vibration, as a the metaphor to help you go beyond rigid thinking. Each word is a code; each word transfers information through frequencies that language itself cannot replicate. This text can never land because it was designed to fly. If you have finished this book, it is because you are ready to be decoded and activated in higher dimensions. Your consciousness understands beyond what your ego can interpret. Nothing you read, regardless of where is written; nothing you hear, regardless of who speaks; should be accepted without careful discernment.

Feel the truth and experience synchronicity in your own essence. Bring it to your heart before you judge. Better, dare to put it in practice and, if it resonates with your essence, embrace it fully. Do not let it pass you by.

> YOU WILL NOT IMPRESS ANYONE IF YOU DECIDE TO GO THIS ROUTE, AND YOU WILL NOT DISAPPOINT ANYONE IF YOU CHOOSE NOT TO. THIS IS A DECISION YOU SHOULD MAKE BASED ON YOUR SPIRITUAL DISCERNMENT, KNOWING NOW WHERE YOU ARE AT THIS TIME ON YOUR OWN PATH.
> Kryon

Appendix

Many thanks to my friend Ernesto Pereira who, on countless occasions in this earthly experience, has been my vehicle for accessing the information I require at the precise moment of synchronicity. The following original papyrus documents are written in the five sacred languages that activate IRB in the DNA. I want to share them with you, dear reader, as they just came to me before this book goes to print. They felt like a master key to open everything to come and everything that has been, at this precise moment: the union of the ancestral and evolution, the sacred and the manifest, the invisible within the visible. I hope you enjoy them as much as I did when Ernesto, with infinite generosity, placed them in my hands.

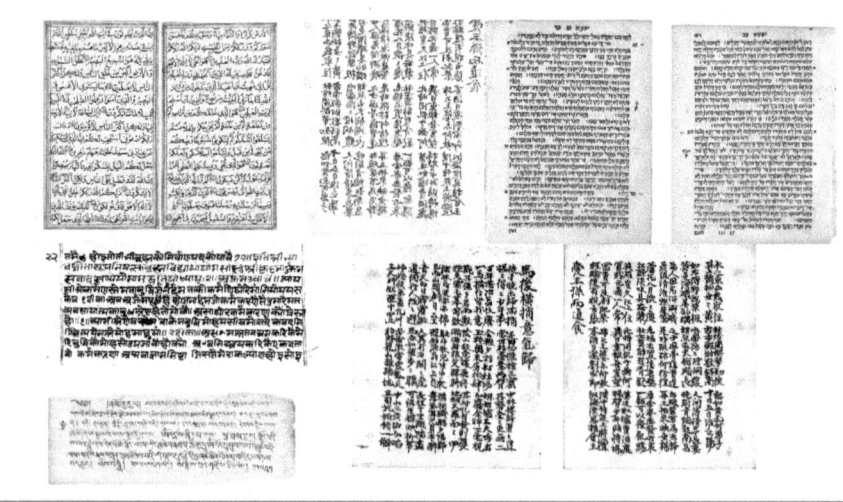

Appendix

1. Egyptian Manuscripts

The Sura, a Qur'an manuscript dating back to the seventeenth century, decorated with gold ink:

2. Hebrew Texts

Bible page from The Tora, printed in Antwerp in 1580:

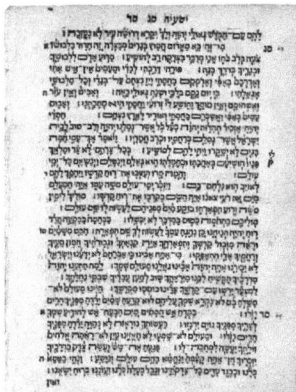

3. Sanskrit Manuscript
Original Manuscript from India, 1850:

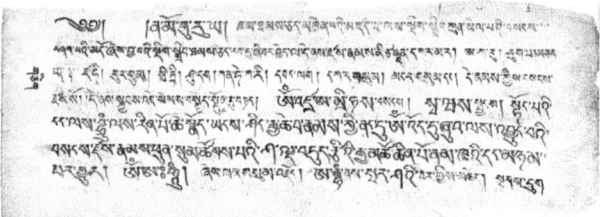

4. Tibetan Manuscripts
Original sacred texts from the eighteenth century:

5. Chinese Texts

Original sacred texts from the eighteenth century:

We close with the last of these treasures. We found part of a Bible page dating back to 1640, describing Aaron's breastplate, decorated with twelve precious gems. It gives us a sign of the arrival of the thirteenth tribe with the thirteenth stone that recognizes IRB in the Cordierite.

Glossary

3D (Abbreviation of Third Density or Third Dimension). The third dimension has hosted human life for millennia. The three-dimensional human energy has a voice, which means it has a language that makes duality viable, encouraging definition through an intellect that defines everything. To define something means to try to understand with the mind what the heart feels, it's to minimize the essence in words and to try to choose between opposing polarities such as *yin* and *yang*, up and down, forward and backward, thick and thin.

Adam Kadmon. The original man, the Universal Man not fallen into sin. The Kabbalists relate this to the ten Sephiroth on the plane of human perception. In the Kabbalah, Adam Kadmon is the manifest Logos, the template for the human being, the ideal man, epitomizing the light body.

Akashic Records. The universal memory of all existence, a multidimensional space where all the experiences of the soul are archived, including the knowledge and experience of past lives, present life and future potentials. This energy system contains all the potentialities that the being, as a spiritual manifestation, possesses for its evolution in this life and true reason to exist. These records exist in the individual, planetary and universal levels, at different vibrational frequencies. In Egypt they are known as the Tablets of Thoth; in the Bible as the Book of Life; in Islam as the Eternal Table, and among the Mayas as the Psi Bank. The adjective Akashic comes from Akasa, a term from the ancient Sanskrit language of India, which means ether, space or the cosmic energy that penetrates the whole universe and is the vehicle that carries sound, light and life.

Amrita. A Sanskrit word that literally means "immortality," often referred to in ancient texts as nectar. Amrita is etymologically related to the Greek ambrosia and carries the same meaning.

Antahkarana. The Antahkarana is an ancient healing and meditation symbol that has been used in Tibet and China for thousands of years, possessing great energetic powers. In Eastern philosophy, is the name given to the bridge that connects the lower mind and the higher mind.

Atman. In Hinduism, Atman is the individual self or the eternal soul, which is identical in essence to Brahman. The core of every person's self is not the body, or the mind, or the ego, but Atman — Soul or Self. Atman is the spiritual essence of all creatures, their innermost essential being. It is essence, it is eternal, it is ageless. Atman is that which lies at the deepest level of one's existence.

Avatar. The Sanskrit word avatar (or avatara) literally means descent. It refers to the descent of divinity from heaven to earth, and is typically used to describe an influential teacher who has marked the history of our planet.

Bardo. A Tibetan word that literally means intermediate state or transitional state. When we transition from one life to another, after we disembody, we stay in the bardo for a time, while we chose our next experience. It is the empty space between thoughts, words, and sensations. It is the stillness that precedes and succeeds every action; the space inhabited by Wisdom, filled with information without interference.

Blueprint. The original Blue plane. It is the spiritual hologram of God. The divine imprint manifested in every being. David Bohm defines it as the implicate order that exists in an unmanifest state and the basis on which all of manifest reality rests.

Chemtrail. A phenomenon consisting of condensation trails that appear in the sky — different from those left by a normal plane. *Chemtrails* are composed of chemicals designed to cause some kind of harm to the population. The term *chemtrail* is an abbreviation of chemical trail.

Christic Race. This refers to the Adamic Race, our race evolved to its highest perfection as Adam Kadmon.

Eons. A measure of time on the geological time scale. It indicates an indefinitely long period, usually much longer than an era.

Gematria. A Kabbalistic method of decoding and interpreting the Torah based on the assignment of numbers to Hebrew letters. Every Hebrew character has a numeric value. When the sum of the numbers making up a word are the same as in another word, one perceives a connection between them, and they are considered together. The word gematria means the geometry of the word. In Judaism, we called this interpretation through the numeric system, the dessert of wisdom.

God. The word that has been assigned to a supreme being considered by monotheistic religions as the creator of the universe. This is a deity that various religions of the world worship and praise. The word comes from the Latin concept deus, capitalized when referring to the aforementioned idea of a supreme being for religions like Christianity, Judaism and Islam. In this book, we use this term to define the human being as a divine particle that comes from the supreme essence but is not separate from its origin.

Holon. Something that is simultaneously a whole and a part. The word was coined by Arthur Koestler in his book The Ghost in the Machine (1967, p. 48).

Any system can be considered a holon, a subatomic particle, and a planet. On the non-physical level, words, ideas, sounds, emotions — everything that can be identified — is simultaneously part of something, and can be viewed as having identical parts of its own. According to American philosopher Ken Wilber, differing from the idea that the cosmos is composed of holons (whole/part), the discovery of what holons share can help us see what evolution has in common with all of its domains: physical, biological, psychological, spiritual, and so on, as well as the guidelines they share.

Indigo Children. An Indigo Child shows special physical, emotional and psychological characteristics different from what is considered "normal.". Too often labeled and medicated as a hyperactive child, he or she possesses extrasensory perception and telekinetic abilities that are generally very poorly documented. Such a child forces sensitive parents to change how they treat and raise him or her, in order to help them to achieve balance and harmony and avoid frustration. No doubt these children are special, and they represent a high percentage of children born in the world today. Indigos are born knowing who they are and what their mission is, so we must respect them for their exceptional qualities and direct them with love, not control. These children show us human evolution; they are smarter than many adults; they come to break from obsolete systems and limiting paradigms. Through IRB, we as adults can ascend to their frequency.

Indigo Ray. This is an organized field of spiritual light that affects the consciousness of Indigo Children and the ultimate transformation of the Earth. When the Indigo Ray comes into balance with the Totality, it allows us to unlearn, freeing ourselves from the barriers set by rules, "I cannots," and fears. This ray awakens us from the hypnotic trance of the destructive hologram so we can build, from consciousness, the hologram in which we remember one hundred percent who we really are in our true magnitude and infinitude, and our purpose for being here. It contains in itself the most occult truths about the universe, God's nature and the Atman destination, among other things. It helps us reveal the hidden keys through which we attain higher power and wisdom. It proclaims the great secrets to all humanity, and its voice resonates clearly for those who want to listen. The Indigo Ray contained within IRB (Indigo Ray Balancing) activates intuition that knows, from the heart, how to make spontaneous decisions that lead to freedom. The Ray is all encompassing and does not identify with anything but moves with the flow of Wisdom. It is a way of being and knowing that language is unable to express. It is acceptance of opposites from neutrality. It is to simply love.

Karma. The word karma means action and mainly refers to the results of physical, verbal and mental acts. Every act leaves a mark or impression that over time produces corresponding results. Our actions are like seeds we plant. Virtuous acts are the seeds of future happiness, and harmful acts are the seeds of future suffering. These seeds produce their effects when they meet the conditions necessary for germination. Further, it may require several lifetimes from the time of the original action until its consequences mature in what we consider linear time.

Koradi Race. The seventh race, to which Indigo Children belong, has come to transform the ego and activate the crystalline and transparent, and to achieve balance between the old and new energy.

Kryon. In the first book channeled by Lee Carroll, Book I, *The End Times*, we are told that Kryon was sent by a group of teachers known as The Brotherhood of Light. Kryon and his group arrived on Earth in 1989 for the Harmonic Convergence, when a measurement of the energy and potential future for humanity was made. As the results were positive, the Kryon group agreed to modify the magnetic grid of the planet to support human enlightenment. Kryon is a being "of magnetic service" and an entity of global service; he has never been human, therefore, he is not an ascended master. More than a "he," Kryon is a consciousness that conveys the concept of unity and wholeness.

Kundalini Energy. Kundalini energy, also known as the power of the serpent, is a portal for raising awareness. Borne of an energetic center located at the base of the spine that awakens and rises up like a snake through all the energy centers of the body, causing changes that promote spiritual evolution. When Kundalini Energy reaches the top of the head, the crown, a unique mystical experience occurs; some have described it as a deep trance state in which connection with the spiritual world occurs.

Lady Gaia. For the Greeks, she was the personification of Earth. This is the great mother, the primitive Greek Mother Goddess, creator and giver of light to Earth and the whole universe. From her union with Uranus (the sky) came the heavenly gods, the Titans and the giants. Her equivalent in the Roman pantheon is Terra. In the new energy, Lady Gaia is the sacred essence of the planet, the living goddess of Earth; she personifies the planet as an instrument of evolution for the current human race.

Merkabah. The *Merkabah* is an interdimensional vehicle represented in isometric form, consisting of three superimposed star tetrahedrons that, when observed, appear to be one. Each of the three is composed of two simple tetrahedrons: the Sun tetrahedron (masculine) pointing up, and the Earth tetrahedron (feminine) pointing down. Each of the star tetrahedrons has a classification and a direction of movement. The first, the female, turns clockwise and the second, the male, turns counter-clockwise. The third is neutral and does not rotate. This is a concept introduced by Drunvalo Melchizedek, and it is considered concrete information on our evolution.

Merkana. In order to evolve toward greater integration of light, the Merkabah is being replaced in the Crystalline Era by the crystalline Mer-Ka-Na. A greater influx of light is taking place on the planet at this time, and this light is coherent and crystalline in nature. Such is the nature of the superior dimensions, which is its true nature. As the crystalline light increases and the energy expands, so does the vehicle of ascension towards a twenty-point star icosahedron.

Metatron's Cube. A quantum accelerator. This figure awakens the electrical laws found in the higher dimensions, as well as processes of transmutation and healing. In sacred geometry, Metatron's Cube is the Fruit of Life, a component of the Flower of Life. It consists of thirteen circles, each one a node that connects to the next by a single straight line, seventy-eight lines in all. Thus, Metatron's Cube is a geometric body directly obtained from the Fruit of Life. Inside the cube are other bodies such as two-dimensional models of all five platonic solids. Metatron's Cube is also considered a sacred glyph and, in the old energy, was drawn around an object or person in order to protect them from demons or satanic powers.

Namaste. The origins of the word Namaste are very remote, as the word comes from the ancient Hindu culture. One of the many languages spoken in India is Sanskrit which, as we have explored in this book, it is one of the sacred languages that open the connection to the infinite information of the Absolute. Hindus use the term *Namaste* as a greeting and a farewell, to give thanks, to ask, or as a sign of respect, usually accompanied by a mudra gesture or joining the palms of the hands in prayer position at the center of the chest.

Namaste is a compound word: namas means greeting or reverence, etymologically related to nam, which means bow down or lean. The suffix te meanwhile is a personal pronoun that means you. Therefore, the most beautiful meaning we can give to this magical word is "The Divine in me honors the Divine in you;" or "I honor the place in you where the entire universe lies;" or "I honor the Light, Love, Truth, Beauty and Peace within you that is also within me, because we are Unity, the same, One." Hereinafter, dear reader, whenever you hear or utter the word Namaste, remember that you are consciously participating in the process of spiritual evolution that this very special word encourages within us.

Parallel Lives. Parallel lives are a phenomenon that has recently received attention thanks to the stories of patients who have undergone the regression therapy of SRT® (Spiritual Response Therapy) of Freedom Healing® and Quantum Synchronization®. The person, through his or her supreme essence or higher self, experiences parallel lives, or the essence of multidimensional souls, in his or her present life and, in some cases, projections of future lives. It is the ability that some human beings possess to recognize that their being or spirit has decided to experience life in simultaneous incarnations.

Physicality. We generally think of knowledge as a body of related facts, and, at the same time, something based in an independent physical reality. Hence, it is natural for us to say, for example, that when we see something red, there is a physical basis for the that. In other words, there must be a physical fact that makes an apple red and not blue. Certainly, viewing things in this simple way is necessary for conversation. Physicality provides a substrate on which to base our interpretations. It is, as Kant would say, a necessary condition for the possibility of perception. Physicality also offers a means of deciding on "correct" interpretations and "misperceptions" concerning our realities.

Power Élite. These are groups of individuals who form secret occult societies, exercising global control over the economic and political spheres. Included in this group are the world's royal families. These groups, which have always exercised their power and control over humanity, are also called the *Illuminati*. David Icke writes about them in more than twenty successful books.

Quantum. In its most essential meaning, Quantum means a whole or partial amount that partially or fully identifies the state of a physical system such as the atom, the atomic nucleus or an elementary particle. When we talk about quantum physics, we refer to the science that studies phenomena from the standpoint of all possibilities; analyzing what is not and explaining phenomena from the perspective of the unseen. Quantum studies observe what is not directly measurable and explains non-intuitive realities such as nonlocality and the indeterminacy of particles. We human beings live in the field of immeasurables; we are part of quantum reality. We belong to the universe. We are made up of atoms with infinite possibilities.

As mentioned in this book, the void is a concept, an idea. The vacuum itself does not exist. Matter is not static, nor predictable. The atom is not a finished permanent reality but is far more malleable than humans think. The empty is merely conceptual and represents all possibilities. Inside the atoms and molecules, matter occupies only one place.

Race. This is not about the present-day races (black, white, et cetera) of humanity but historical stages in human evolution. Not about racial discrimination, genetic alterations, hybridizations or crossbreeding, this deals with the term root races as specified by H. P. Blavatzky as follows:

The first root race was the Polarian, whose individuals were fully awake and had divine ethereal bodies; they lived in the ancient continent of Thule, situated at the current northern polar cap.

The second root race was the Hyperborean, the original inhabitants of Europe.

The third root race was made up of the inhabitants of the continent Lemuria, also known as Mu; this would have been the race in which man materialized completely.

The fourth root race consisted of the inhabitants of Atlantis, the hypothetical lost continent par excellence; those people were tall and divided into two sexes. This advanced civilization gave rise to present-day humans.

The fifth root race is the present humanity, subdivided into the races we know so well.

The sixth and seventh root races represent advanced stages of the current root race, more ethereal, beginning with the Indigo Children.

Sefirot. According to the Kabbalah, the sefirot (the plural is sefirá, which means numbers in the Hebrew language) means the ten emanations of God through which the world was created. According to Kabbalistic tradition, Yahweh contracted his infinite light in what it is called in Hebrew tsimtsum and created the sefirá.

Shaman. A person with the ability to alter reality, or our collective perception of reality. Shamans are not bound to causal logic. This can be expressed as, for example, the faculty of healing and communicating with spirits. Shamans possess visionary and divining skills and are usually tribal elders who carry forward ancestral traditions.

Tamera. An intentional community and peace research center founded in 1995 on a farm of 150 hectares near Colos, Portugal. There nearly 160 people live and study. Their goal is to become "a self-sufficient, sustainable and duplicable communitarian model for

Glossary

nonviolent cooperation and cohabitation among humans, animals, nature, and Creation, for a future of peace for all."

Tetragrammaton. This represents the sacred name of God contained within mantra twelve of IRB, one of three that activates the fourth Nuclear Command. The four Hebrew letters YHWH or JHVH that form the biblical proper name of God, are read from right to left. It is interpreted in many religions as Jehovah, Yahweh or Yaweh. We could also translate it as to become, or the reason to become, or the Existing One, or the I Am. This implies compliance with a defined purpose for the good of humanity. That is why it is called "the God of all the earth" (Genesis 17:1) and not just of Israel. This Hebrew symbol looks like this:

This expresses the domination of spirit over the elements of nature — earth, air, fire and water — and is represented as a flaming five-pointed star:

יהוה

The Book of Knowledge: The Keys of Enoch®. The Keys of Enoch is a para-physical codebook written in 1973 by Dr. J.J. Hurtak. It is a text of higher-consciousness experiences that explain how the

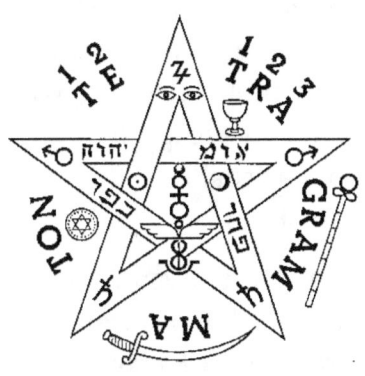

human race is connected to the higher evolutionary structure of universal intelligence. The connection is established through sixty-four areas concerning future science, a continuous human development program covering a broad spectrum of independent scientific confirmations. This book is meant to prepare us for the paradigm shift that will affect all aspects of the social, psychological and spiritual dimensions of earthly life.

The Secret Doctrine. This is a book, or rather a collection of several volumes, that synthesize science, religion and philosophy. One of the main works of Helena Blavatsky, it talks about the scientific, philosophical and religious thought of the day. The first volume was titled Cosmogenesis (1888), consisting mainly of studies concerning the evolution of the universe. The second volume is Anthropogenesis. The two volumes represent a summary of Theosophy, a movement founded by Blavatsky and directed by Osho for over twenty years. The Theosophical Society published a third volume after the death of Blavatsky, including a collection of his articles. These are the titles of the six volumes: Cosmogenesis; Universal Archaic Symbolism; Anthropogenesis; The Archaic Symbolism of the World Religions and Science; Science, Religion and Philosophy; The Object of the Mysteries, and The Practice Of Occult Philosophy.

The Wheel of Samsara. This refers to the concept of reincarnation in the philosophical traditions of India: Hinduism, Buddhism and Jainism. It corresponds to the suffering of reincarnated beings trying to liberate themselves by way of enlightenment, or nirvana. The time needed to escape from samsara depends on the person's dedication to spiritual practices and the weight of karma accumulated in previous lives.

Thoth. It is said that Thoth was an Atlantean priest-king who founded a colony in ancient Egypt after the sinking of the mother country; also, he built the Great Pyramid of Giza, which historically has been attributed to Cheops. In this pyramid was incorporated Thoth's knowledge of ancient wisdom, where he stored the records and instruments of Atlantis. For about 16,000 years, he ruled the ancient civilization of Egypt. At that time, Egypt was a barbaric society which then evolved to a high degree of civilization. Thoth was immortal; he had conquered death. His vast wisdom made him ruler of the various post-Atlantean colonies, including those of South and Central America. When the time came to leave Egypt, he erected the great pyramid over the entrance of the Great Halls of Amenti, where he stored his records and appointed guards from among the highest of his people, to watch over his secrets.

Threefold Flame. The threefold flame, or divine spark, is the seed of the divine within the human being. It is the seed of the inner Christ and inner Buddha. The threefold flame is represented in the heart chakra, embodying the same qualities of love, wisdom and power manifested in divinity, in the heart of the Presence — the I am — and in the heart of the Higher Self. This divine spark is the passport to immortality.

UFO. Unidentified Flying Object.

Yin-Yang. This is a dynamic symbol that shows the continuing interaction and balance of two opposing energies. A symbol that expresses harmony, the *yin-yang* circle expresses equality and embraces the opposites that create the greater whole. Without the yin, the yang cannot exist and vice versa; without the interaction of the two, there is no generation of life. There is no opposition between *yin* and *yang*, as they complement each other. In the Tao Te Ching, Lao Tzu wrote, "Everything has inside both the yin and yang, and from their alternate ascent and descent, new life is born." When one of the two energies reaches its maximum expression, a transformation begins in its opposite; this is what the two oppositely colored eyes in the image represent. At its maximum expression, the yang contains the seed of the yin, and the yin contains the seed of the yang. The yin is the feminine principle, meaning intuition, earth, darkness, passivity and absorption. *Yang is the male principle, incorporating heaven, light, action and penetration.* We could conclude then that this symbol represents the generating principle of all things, from the primordial sources from which they arise.

For more information, gifts and experiences from
IRB – Transforming Fear Into Love
visit:
bit.ly/XimenaDuqueValencia_IRB

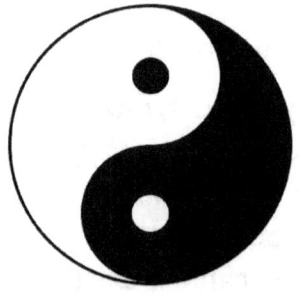

References

BACKSTER, C. (2003). *Primary Perception.* Anza, CA, EE. UU.: White Rose Millenium Press.

BENÍTEZ, J. J. (2011). *Caballo de Troya 9. Caná.* España: Planeta.

BLAVATSKY, H. P. (1888). *La doctrina secreta.* Buenos Aires, Argentina: Kier.

BRAUD, W. y SCHLITZ, M. (1997). Distant intentionality and healing: assessing the evidence. *Alternative Terapies,* 3(6), 62-73.

CARROLL, L. (2010). *Kryon XII: Las doce capas del ADN. Un estudio esotérico de la Maestría interior.* España: Vésica Piscis.

CARROLL, L. y TOBER, J. (2001). *Los niños índigo: un libro especial para los que tienen hijos pequeños hiperactivos o con déficit de atención.* Barcelona, España: Obelisco.

COLLINS, S. (2008). *Los juegos del hambre.* EE. UU.: Scholastic Press.

DUHM, D. (2012). *The sacred matrix.* Berghoff, Monika, u. Saskia Breithart: Verlag Meiga.

GARCÍA, J. C. *Los cuentos de hadas en el cine.* Recuperado de http://www.juancarlosgarciaweb.com/biografia_frame.html

GOETNEICK AMBROSE, S. (septiembre de 2004). Cell *Decision.* The Dallas Morning News.

HALL, J. (2007). *La biblia de los cristales.* Madrid, España: Gaia.

HANCOCK, G. (1995). *Finger Prints of the Gods.* Nueva York, EE. UU.: Three Rivers Press.

HAWKS, J. (s.f.). *Paleoanthropology, genetics, and evolution.* Recuperado de http:/johnhawks.net

HOWARD, P. (1999). *The Owner's Manual for the Brain.* Atlanta, EE. UU.: Bard Press.

HURTAK, J. J. (1977). *El Libro del Conocimiento: Las Claves de Enoc.* Los Gatos, CA: EE. UU.: The Academy For Future Science.

HURTAK, J. J. (2005). *Los 72 nombres de Dios.* Los Gatos, CA: EE. UU.: The Academy for Future Science.

ICKE, D. (2009). *Dejando ir el miedo.* (Conferencia). Melbourne, Australia: Recuperado de http://www.youtube.com/watch?v=u43r9F2sVpw

ICKE, D. (2011). *El mayor secreto: el libro que cambiará el mundo.* Barcelona, España: Obelisco.

ICKE, D. (2013). *La conspiración mundial y cómo acabar con ella.* Barcelona, España: Obelisco.

LIPTON, B. (2005). *The Biology of Belief.* California, EE. UU.: Elite Books.

LIPTON, B. y BHAERMAN, S. (2009). *Spontaneous Evolution: Our Positive Future and How to Get There from Here.* California, EE. UU.: Hay House.

MAJOR JENKINS, J. y MATZ, M. (2005). *El códice azteca: la iniciación espiritual de la pirámide de fuego.* Barcelona, España: Minotauro.

MCTAGGART, L. (2006). *El campo, en busca de la fuerza secreta que mueve el universo.* España: Sirio.

MONTAGNIER, L. (2009). *Las batallas de la vida: más vale prevenir que curar.* Madrid, España: Alianza.

PALMER HALL, M. (1928). *The Secret Teaching of All Ages: An Encyclopedic Outline of Masonic, Hermetic, Qabbalistic and Rosicrucian Symbolical*

Philosophy. San Francisco, EE. UU.: H. S. Crocker.

RAMTHA, J. (2003). *The mistery of Birth and Death. Redefining the Self.* EE. UU.: Arkano Books.

SHERMAN, H. (1988). *Conozca su propia mente.* México: Diana.

STRASSMAN, R. (2001). *DMT. La molécula espiritual.* Rochester, Vermont, EE. UU.: Park Street Press.

TALBOT, M. (2007). *El universo holográfico: una visión nueva y extraordinaria de la realidad.* Madrid, España: Palmyra.

TOLLE, E. (2005). *Una nueva Tierra. Un despertar al propósito de su vida.* Colombia: Norma.

WILCOCK, D. (2011). *The Source Field Investigations.* EE. UU.: Penguin.

WINTER, D. (2002). *Psicogeometría.* Argentina: Kier.

www.ingramcontent.com/pod-product-compliance
Lightning Source LLC
Chambersburg PA
CBHW070223190526

45169CB00001B/61